Healing Digestive Disorders

Natural Treatments for Gastrointestinal Conditions

Third Edition

Andrew Gaeddert

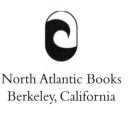

North Atlantic Books
Berkeley, California

Published by

North Atlantic Books   Get Well Foundation
P.O. Box 12327   8001A Capwell Drive
Berkeley, California 94712   Oakland, California 94621

Cover and book design by Catherine E. Campaigne
Copyediting by Nissi Wang

Printed in the United States of America

Healing Digestive Disorders: Natural Treatments for Gastrointestinal Conditions, Third Edition is sponsored by the Society for the Study of Native Arts and Sciences, a nonprofit educational corporation whose goals are to develop an educational and cross-cultural perspective linking various scientific, social, and artistic fields; to nurture a holistic view of arts, sciences, humanities, and healing; and to publish and distribute literature on the relationship of mind, body, and nature.

Healing Digestive Disorders: Natural Treatments for Gastrointestinal Conditions, Third Edition is also sponsored by the Get Well Foundation, a nonprofit organization whose purpose is to educate the public and health care providers about natural therapies that are complements to Western medicine. Get Well Foundation operates a clinic, publishes books, and sponsors seminars.

North Atlantic Books' publications are available through most bookstores. For further information, call 800-733-3000 or visit our website at www.northatlanticbooks.com.

MEDICAL DISCLAIMER: The following information is intended for general information purposes only. Individuals should always see their health care provider before administering any suggestions made in this book. Any application of the material set forth in the following pages is at the reader's discretion and is his or her sole responsibility.

New ISBN: 978-1-55643-743-4
New Publication: 2008

The Library of Congress has cataloged the earlier editions as follows:

Gaeddert, Andrew.
   Healing digestive disorders : natural treatments for gastrointestinal conditions / by Andrew Gaeddert.-2nd ed.
      p.   cm.
   Includes bibliographical references and index.
   ISBN 1-55643-508-8 (pbk.)
      1. Digestive organs—Diseases—Alternative treatment. 2. Naturopathy. 3. Medicine, Chinese.   4. Herbs—Therapeutic use. [DNLM: 1. Gastrointestinal Diseases—therapy—Popular Works.   2. Complementary Therapies—Popular Works.   3. Medicine, Herbal—Popular Works. WI 140 G127h 2004]   I. Title.
   RC802.G25 2004
   616.3'3-dc22   2004000096

1   2   3   4   5   6   DATA   12   11   10   09   08

Acknowledgments

I would like to give special thanks to Lou Ann Gaeddert, Carol Eckels, Patricia Puckett, Michael Clauson, and Nissi Wang.

Table of Contents

Introduction
to the Third Edition

S ince the publication of the first edition of *Healing Digestive Disorders,* I continue to help the countless number of clients who make appointments at our clinic wanting help with their digestive disorders. There are two types of people requesting help. Those I call the *believers* and the *visitors.*

Believers are willing to do whatever it takes. They follow instructions about herbs to use, and also follow through on dietary and lifestyle suggestions. They realize that conventional Western medicine does not offer lasting solutions for gastrointestinal conditions, and are willing to be patient with natural therapies.

On the other hand, the *visitors* may want to improve their health. They may be voracious readers, and may experiment with various approaches; however, the *visitors* usually have preconceived notions about how they "ought" to be treated, and how they "should" progress. The *visitors* take the herbs and supplements, but expect results to be as immediate as they are with prescription drugs. There are excuses why they did not follow the recommended regimen of herbs, or follow through with a dietary and exercise program. Much of their time is spent wondering why they were singled out for digestive disorders.

While it is true that there is a genetic predisposition for digestive disorders, they do not happen arbitrarily. Almost all digestive disorders are triggered by stress, improper food, and sometimes a toxin. For example, a typical ulcer patient usually does not take the time to plan healthy meals, exercise, and participate in a personal stress reduction program.

Natural therapies are gentle to the system but take longer to act than drugs or surgery. The benefit of adopting healthy habits and using natural therapies is that it is possible to achieve lasting relief for all your symptoms and prevent new disorders from occurring.

For example, one of our clients, Dorothy, came to us with irritable bowel syndrome, chronic fatigue, and dry skin. By faithfully sticking to our recommended protocol for one year, she was able to eliminate all her symptoms. And using natural therapies, she did not fall into the trap of using drugs to correct drug side effects.

Before he came to our clinic, Steve ate antacids by the handful. After a short period of time the antacids stopped working. His doctor prescribed an acid blocker. From the medication he noticed increased diarrhea, which was treated with antibiotics. After several courses of antibiotics, he ended up with a fungal infection from all the antibiotics. The result was a liver reaction to the antifungal drug and hospitalization. We find this pattern in our clinic quite often from those people who are not willing to make the time and effort to eat healthy foods, exercise, and use stress reduction techniques.

It is understandable that people are skeptical about alternative medicine. The practitioner may not wear a white coat, and may not have an office in the medical building. The credentials of an acupuncturist or herbalist may not be understood. More-over, it may not be understood that dietary supplements such as Chinese herbal formulas are regulated and are safer than conventional foods. Over the years, medical industry safety issues for herbs have been called into question by the media; however, herbs have been used for centuries, and as a result, one could argue that more is known about their safety than drugs, which have only been around for decades or less.

The best way to start using natural therapies is to find a practitioner you are comfortable with and who has experience treating your particular condition. It is essential that you communicate with your practitioner. Once you find a person you trust, it is important to follow his or her directions exactly. We find that many of the *visitors* are constantly tweaking their program and taking too few tablets, or skipping days. This compromises results and delays the healing process.

Who do you know that has used natural methods successfully? Is there a way you can reach out to that person? Having a buddy or sponsor is useful to keep you on track, and helps support you if you get discouraged. The journey to good health need not be a painful journey, yet it is not always a straight line. There may be days when you feel 100 percent, followed by a day when you feel you have made no progress at all. As mentioned in the text, it is very important for you to keep a journal to help chart your progress. And it is important that you acknowledge to yourself any progress that you make.

Mary, who elected not to get gastrointestinal surgery, was discouraged because her friend Karen, who had the surgery, was much better and not having symptoms. However, Karen ended up having complications due to the surgery and nearly died. Mary was not able to visualize being healed and was not able to see the progress she had made; instead she compared herself to Karen and stopped the program. It is crucial that you not compare yourself to others. Instead, visualize how you will feel when you are healed and celebrate the progress you make.

What can you do in order to become a *believer* rather than a *visitor?* What beliefs would be important for your ongoing healing? Important beliefs may be: *I will follow my practitioner's advice faithfully. I will trust my own experience about natural healing methods. I am worth healing.*

Chapter One

My Personal Story

When I was 19, I almost died of Crohn's disease, an inflammatory disorder of the intestines. I had eaten at a restaurant where it seems I contracted food poisoning. Shortly after the meal my main symptoms were abdominal cramping, fever, and diarrhea. When I did not feel better after two days, I went to the health clinic at the university I attended. I was prescribed Valium, a sedative, and told to take hot baths and Tylenol. Even several days on this regimen proved ineffective, and by this time I felt very weak. I took a cab to the emergency room, but the doctors said there was nothing they could do, that the condition would improve on its own. After a few more days of terrible shooting abdominal pains, diarrhea, fever, inability to keep food down, and weakness, I was finally admitted to the hospital.

Once there, my condition worsened. My temperature soared to 106°F (41°C). I was put into intensive isolation; anyone entering the room had to put on a disposable gown, mask, hat, and surgical gloves. These articles ended up in a hall receptacle, eventually to be burned.

A high-tech machine was unsuccessful in lowering my body temperature. As a last ditch effort, I received alcohol rubdowns in order to reduce my temperature. My only nutrition was received through a tube. I was injected with intravenous antibiotics as well as with Valium every four hours. Finally, with rest, my condition slowly improved. After innumerable tests it was finally pronounced that I was suspected of having Crohn's disease. The next month I spent at home recuperating, eating a limited-fiber diet, and taking vitamins and antibiotics.

My parents had always said that I was "the kid with the cast-iron stomach." They felt they were getting their money's worth whenever they took me to an all-you-can-eat restaurant, since I was very active and could put away great quantities of food. My favorite food at that time was roast beef. I can remember going to a restaurant that offered unlimited roast beef. I ate, went for a run in the parking lot to work up more appetite, and ate some more!

As a teenager, I became aware of a sensitivity to spaghetti, another one of my favorite foods. Sometimes I could eat spaghetti with tomato sauce and not have any symptoms, while other times I got gas pains. It was not until I was in college that I realized I had chronic digestive symptoms. Looking back, it is easy to diagnose the sources of my problems: stress, lack of exercise, and the college cafeteria.

In terms of stress, at that time I was experiencing great personal turmoil. I was three thousand miles away from my family in a new town where I did not have many friends. I had just finished a job as a counselor to abused and emotionally disturbed children, an experience that brought me joy and satisfaction, but was also traumatic. I was enrolled in college, but my grades were not good enough for the graduate school that I wanted to attend.

As for exercise, what little I did get was even stressful. I was one of the only white basketball players in my neighborhood and was often heckled with racial slurs and called "the blind man," because I wore glasses. Although in high school I had been an athlete and played on several varsity teams, meaning that I got some sort of daily exercise, I was not skilled enough to make the college basketball team. Rather than continue to exercise, even just for fun, I figured my studies were more important.

Diet was another cause of my digestive problems. After I moved away from home the quality of my diet deteriorated. The main entrées in the college cafeteria were either not appetizing or were loaded with grease. Not surprisingly, fat and grease can contribute to digestive conditions. I was also trying to be a vegetarian and was eating many foods that were not good for me. I used soy and cheese as my main sources of protein, both of which are common allergens. Allergens can cause inflammatory conditions to flare up.

Because I was away from home, for the first time I could indulge in sweets. Excess sweets are another major dietary cause of digestive disorders, as is alcohol. At that time, I also started to drink. Unlimited alcohol was available at parties each weekend, and I often had beer a few days a week while socializing with friends or watching sports events on TV.

Finally, another contributing factor to my digestive problems was that I continued to drink milk. I now believe that humans should stop drinking milk at age eighteen or younger (see "Lactose Intolerance" section, Chapter Four). Anyone with a digestive condition should stop regardless of age. No wonder I felt like I had an active volcano in my stomach, and why I prayed for relief.

When my problems first developed I had gone to the university health clinic. I was examined and was told it was my nerves; I received a prescription for the sedative phenobarbital. I was referred to the school psychologist, who told me, "Your stomach isn't messed up, you are."

In the year before my admission to the hospital, I had gotten sick more than usual (due to the above habits, no doubt) and had taken several courses of antibiotics. Antibiotics destroy the friendly bacteria in the intestinal tract as well as the disease-causing ones. The resulting imbalance may have been another contributing cause of my symptoms. I was next referred to a gastroenterologist who administered a barium enema. He said that I was not intolerant to milk, that there was nothing wrong except that I had a "spastic colon." He prescribed a fiber product, which only made my symptoms worse. One night after eating a spaghetti dinner, the tearing abdominal pains forced me to the local emergency room. My stomach was pumped, and though weak, I felt much better the next day.

During part of this time I was living in rural Mendocino County in California. It was rumored that the water was bad and many of my neighbors either boiled their drinking water or drank bottled water; I took no such precautions since there was no formal decree. Later, when I frequently suffered bouts of stomach flu–like symptoms, I began to believe that I had contracted a parasitic infection through drinking the infected water. Parasitic infections are a common cause of digestive problems (see "Parasites" section, Chapter Four).

I also suffered from terrible hayfever in the spring and summer. That year, I read a book about natural treatments for hayfever. At the suggestion of this book, I stopped drinking milk, even though my doctor had said I was not milk intolerant. My digestive and allergy symptoms did in fact improve, but other remedies I tried from health food stores didn't seem to help.

After graduating from college, I went to live in San Francisco. One of my jobs was selling an ancient Tibetan herbal remedy to health food stores and alternative doctors. The remedy had been studied in clinical trials in Europe, although the U.S. Food and Drug Administration had not approved it for sale in the U.S. This exposure to alternative medicines opened up a new world to me. I also began to learn about Chinese herbs. I tried them during the periods when I had flare-ups. Since being hospitalized initially, I still had several flare-ups a year, during which I experienced severe pain and had to eat a bland diet. Much of the rest of the time I had frequent gas, abdominal bloating, and a feeling of fullness. I found that by taking a Chinese herbal remedy, I was able to reduce the flare-ups to two or three days instead of the usual two weeks. I also found Chinese herbal decoctions (herbs boiled to make a tea) gave me the energy to recover from colds and flu.

These experiences lead me to study all I could about herbal medicine. I developed a passion for Chinese herbs, introducing doctors, health food stores, and individuals to herbal medicine. Testimonials from doctors and herbalists, whose patients used these products, began coming into the office where I worked. After this company folded, demand for our herbal remedies remained. I decided to start my own company manufacturing Chinese and Western herbal products, slowly adding more and more formulas to my line.

These early days were very trying. I faced a vendetta by a federal government employee who seemed to consider my demise a way of boosting his career. Luckily his actions were so outrageous, such as sending an unapproved and slanderous questionnaire to my customers, that my congressman took an interest and helped resolve this situation. During my tribulations, I kept my goal in mind: to help the millions of people who have digestive, gynecological, and immune disorders by publicizing, researching, and writing about the benefits of herbal medicine. The herbal formulas that I have developed have now been successfully used by thousands of digestive patients. Several of the formulas have been researched at prestigious universities such as the University of California, San Francisco.

Fortunately, in the last ten years, herbal medicines have moved from the health food fringe movement into the aisles of major drug store chains. Consumers and even medical professionals are now more open to their use. When I went to my ear, nose, and throat doctor even she extolled the benefits of two popular herbs, echinacea and ginkgo!

Many people ask me about the current state of my Crohn's disease. In the past ten years I have had only one serious flare-up. It was brought on by eating popcorn, a food my body does not tolerate. Luckily, herbal remedies rapidly resolved that flare-up. I have never been on steroids, a common treatment for Crohn's. For this, I am very grateful. I quickly resolve any abdominal bloating or intestinal gas I experience by being more careful about what I eat and by taking herbal remedies. I also have come to understand that antioxidant vitamins and folic acid have a preventive effect on inflammatory mechanisms. I take these on a daily basis. In order to avoid antibiotics, which for me cause an exacerbation of digestive symptoms, I treat any cold or flu with herbs. Finally, I remain committed to exercise, daily meditation, and my mission of helping people with digestive and other disorders.

What I Have Done For Myself You Can Too

Conventional medicine does not have much to offer an individual with a chronic digestive problem. Doctors can turn off an inflammatory reaction with drugs, repair physical damage, or remove a diseased organ. However, there is little they can do to restore normal health. You can do this yourself with the methods suggested in this book. Even if you cannot attain perfect health, you can at least improve your level of health. It is likely you can reduce the use of medications and avoid their side effects by following the herbal and dietary supplement protocols and lifestyle adjustments described herein. Genes may predispose you to a digestive disorder; however, it is your lifestyle that determines whether you control your digestive disorder or your digestive disorder controls you. Here are the general areas you will need to address.

Stress Reduction

In working with digestive clients for more than ten years, I have noticed that most people with digestive disorders are poor adapters to stress. People with digestive disorders are likely to have a flare-up of their disease during, after, or in anticipation of a stressful event. Friends or colleagues facing the same situation may have no physical symptoms, or may develop shoulder and neck tension, a headache, or come down with a cold or the flu, rather than a digestive disorder. Those with chronic problems of the digestive tract tend to hold their tension there.

Even if you have been given a set of genes that make your abdomen seem like a minefield, you can reduce your symptoms with stress reduction exercises and activities. Digestive problems tend to run in families. If you have a digestive disorder, it is likely that another member of your family has one also, even if it has a different medical name. In my own family, my aunt has Crohn's disease, my dad has had gastric ulcers. Other family members have problems such as constipation, nervous stomach, or intolerance to fats, which have not required a medical diagnosis. Therefore, being born with a predisposition toward digestive problems does not mean that you cannot control it, in part with stress reduction.

Diet

Essential to changing your digestive health is changing your diet. Some of the suggestions in this book, such as avoiding milk, are well documented in the medical literature. Others are based on the experience of practitioners, ranging from traditional herbalists to modern allergy specialists. I have developed a daily digestive diet that will help you identify trigger foods, that is, foods that don't agree with your system and cause symptoms or flareups. Once you learn what your trigger foods are, and after a period of elimination, you can usually eat small amounts of the desired foods on an occasional basis. Products that I am sensitive to are beets, raw vegetables, and juices. I like the taste of beets, and can eat small amounts occasionally without suffering diarrhea. I can tolerate salads only when seasoned with black pepper, and when they have minimal amounts of dressing.

Another dietary area of consideration is the underlying temperature of your constitution—hot or cold. This determines which foods you can tolerate and which you must eat with caution. My own constitution is cold, so the warming black pepper counterbalances the cooling effect of the raw vegetables. If the weather is especially cold and damp and my digestive system is not functioning optimally, I only eat cooked vegetables. I've found that most vegetable and fruit juices do not agree with my system. Above all, I have found through years of practice that the best diet for me is the one I was raised on, namely meat, fish, soup, vegetables, fresh fruit, and some sort of starch. However, for someone with a hot constitution it may be more appropriate to eat more cooling fruit and raw vegetables, less meat. Ultimately, through trial and error you must identify which foods are problematic for you. The effort will be well worth it.

Acceptance and Reconciliation

For myself, a change of attitude was as important as a change of diet. Digestive symptoms are part of the body's warning system. Just like a burglar alarm that makes loud noises when there is an unwanted intruder, your body gives you a signal when you have introduced something that is unwanted and continues giving you warning signals until you stop. Instead of countering the symptoms, take them as guides in your detective work to discover what is bothering you. In this book I offer several exercises to determine possible causes of your digestive symptoms.

For a long time I lamented the fact that I couldn't eat certain foods and drink alcohol. Now, I have not only accepted these limitations, but I see their good aspects. For example, by reducing my alcohol intake I am protecting my liver and digestive system. After quitting regular drinking for thirty days, I realized that some of my headaches and digestive problems were due to alcohol. Clearly, I didn't need it. I may still choose to drink or eat foods I am sensitive to, but now I know how to moderate their effects with herbs and other dietary supplements. The only food I have had to eliminate completely is popcorn, which invariably wreaks havoc on my system no matter what precautions I take.

The strength of this book is that it is not a medical book. The suggestions put forward are meant to be a complement to, not a substitute for, your medical doctor's instructions and your own "gut feelings." In the next section, I'll introduce quick tips you can implement to eliminate or avoid digestive symptoms.

Why I Use Chinese Medicine

The Chinese have a very old culture. They have been using herbal remedies for thousands of years. The first medical text was written about two thousand years ago and it is still used by students of Chinese medicine. In the U.S., over one million patients use acupuncture and Chinese herbs each year.

In China, the most common treatments for digestive disorders are herbs and nutritional therapy. Hospital studies have been conducted proving that appropriately administered herbs can even circumvent gastrointestinal surgeries in many cases.

Chinese tradition views digestive patients according to their condition or temperature. Haven't you met people who run hot, or boil over at the slightest insult? Don't you know people who are always cold, when others are warm? Chinese medicine takes these constitutional factors into account before prescribing herbs or making dietary recommendations. Foods, as well as people, can be similarly classified. For example, chili peppers are warming and ice cream is cooling. According to traditional Chinese medicine, people with digestive disorders should not consume foods or beverages colder than room temperature. This means no iced drinks and iced foods, nor should drinks or food be eaten right out of the refrigerator. Raw foods, such as salad, should be consumed cautiously when the weather is cold, and never during flare-ups. Fried foods should be avoided.

Chinese herbalists even caution us to dress appropriately. Wearing skimpy clothing can subject one to drafts. This leads to poor circulation, which interferes with digestion and other processes.

As examples of the above principles of Chinese medicine, take the following two individuals: William, a 24-year-old college student and athlete who has Crohn's disease, gets entirely different herbs than Grace, a frail 85-year-old grandmother who has the same disease. William has what is considered a hot condition. He complains of fevers, bloodshot eyes, and shooting abdominal pain. Grace feels cold and tired all the time and has diarrhea; she is said to have a cold condition. I recommended that William take herbs that had cooling, and pain relieving properties. He was advised to abstain from alcohol and spicy food. I also suggested that he not train so vigorously, to prevent exhaustion. I recommended that he drink peppermint tea (hot or at room temperature), as it has antispasmodic properties. Grace was counseled to take warming herbs, as well as to eat and drink everything hot. I also recommended ginger tea, which has warming properties.

Below is a chart for you to assess your basic constitution; dietary and lifestyle suggestions are also included.

Cold Condition

A person with many of the following symptoms is considered to have a cold pattern and should be treated accordingly.

- Cold hands and feet (can also be due to liver pattern)
- Cold lower back
- Low energy
- No desire
- Fearful
- Frequent urination
- Feels better in the summer
- Rarely sweats
- Loose stools (can also be due to heat)
- Weak voice
- No desire to drink
- Clear or white phlegm
- Lack of appetite
- Clear urine
- Dizziness
- Edema
- Delayed menstruation, pale menstrual blood

Pulse:	Sinking, slow
Tongue:	Pale or white coating
Limit:	Intake of dairy products
	Intake of salads or uncooked foods
	Never use ice

Emphasize:

Meats:	Beef or chicken soup
Teas:	Ginger
	Cinnamon
	Cloves
	Chinese ginseng
Spices:	Nutmeg
	Garlic (if no sensitivity)
	Black pepper
	Fennel
	Orange or tangerine peel (in tea or soups)
Lifestyle Tips:	Always dress warmly especially in winter
	Eat everything hot
	Try to get daily exercise to improve your circulation

Hot Condition

A person with many of the following symptoms is considered to have a hot pattern, and should be treated accordingly.

- Feels warm all over
- Frequently thirsty
- Smokes
- Feels stress, anxiety
- Easily angered

- Constipation (can also be due to cold)
- Athletic
- Feels better in winter
- Sweats a lot
- Prone to afternoon slump
- Dark urine
- Loud voice
- Dominating, aggressive
- Easily upset
- Overly emotional
- Irritable
- Dry cough
- Yellow phlegm
- Thin
- Early and heavy menstruation, bright red blood
- Insomnia

Pulse:	Rapid
Tongue:	Red, or sticky yellow coating
Limit:	Spicy food, alcohol, coffee Salads and other raw foods during flare-ups Avoid fried foods Take care not to get too hot or exhausted in the spring and summer

Emphasize:

Vegetables:	Vegetable soups Cucumber, cooked cabbage, cooked greens
Teas:	Peppermint, chamomile, dandelion, chrysanthemum, red raspberry leaf American ginseng
Spices:	Seaweed Orange or tangerine peel (in tea or soups)

Lifestyle Tips: Try to engage in daily meditation or prayer as well as exercise

Summary

In this chapter I have discussed the most important aspects of digestive healing: stress reduction, avoiding trigger foods and beverages, accepting limitations, and enjoying life. In the following chapters I provide a multifaceted, natural approach to the identification and treatment of various digestive disorders.

Chapter Two has tips for reducing digestive symptoms and achieving better health. Chapter Three provides more detailed information about natural remedies used in the treatment of digestive disorders. Chapter Four contains an alphabetical listing of disorders and corresponding natural therapies, as well as case studies that highlight the particular disorder and typical courses of treatment. Chapter Five includes a diet plan that has proven helpful to thousands of people.

Chapter Two

Tips and Affirming Changes

Decide to Heal

Do you really want to heal? I had a client named Candide. On the surface she led a perfect life: She had a job she liked, even though she admitted it was stressful; a beautiful house; a loving family. Candide had gone to many health professionals, but none of them had been able to help her chronic constipation and abdominal bloating. She had tried many diets, dozens of supplements, all without results. Although she had dabbled with a variety of techniques, she undertook none of them wholeheartedly, always saying that her life was too stressful to make the required commitment to change. She was not able to follow through with the simplest requests. For instance, I mentioned that taking a bath before bedtime would help her insomnia (and help her get off the sleeping pills that were causing the constipation and bloating), but she claimed that she was too busy. Similarly, I recommended that every day she take a thermos of chamomile tea to work and drink it, but she did not like the flavor, or the alternatives I presented. Finally, I mentioned that she should make it a point to exercise every day. She said that she had tried aerobics, but it had hurt her joints. I encouraged Candide to at least walk every day and she concurred, telling me she had to walk the dog anyway. So we agreed that she would walk the dog for a half an hour each day. But in the end even following *this* suggestion was too much; there was never the time, her family needed her.

Perhaps getting sick was the only attention she felt she deserved. Not surprisingly, she cancelled her third appointment because "a conflict had arisen."

In contrast to Candide, Debbie, with a several year history of digestive disorders, came in with the attitude, "I'll do whatever it takes!" In our first session we discussed the importance of eating regular meals, especially breakfast. She was willing to take both herbal teas and tablets, which had immediate benefits. She employed several of the lifestyle tips I suggested (mentioned later in this chapter). She was able to incorporate the ones that helped her the most into her daily regime.

Within a month she was eating more regularly, had significantly less abdominal pain, and was walking every day and practicing yoga. With the help of the digestive clearing diet, she was able to identify problem foods. In time she was able to reduce, then eliminate the pharmaceutical medication she was taking, which had caused unpleasant side effects. In this short period, she was no longer constantly worried about her digestion.

If you, like Debbie, are willing to make dietary and lifestyle changes, the benefits are limitless.

Visualize Yourself as Being Healthy

If you want to heal your digestive system, it is imperative to look toward a future in which you have no digestive problems. As motivational speaker Anthony Robbins says, "Your past does not equal your future." The more positive you feel about your future, the better your digestion will be able to work, since worry and discontent no longer block it.

Ralph Waldo Emerson, the great American writer, said, "A man is what he thinks about all day long." It is important that you anticipate a future that is productive for yourself and others. All too often those of us with a chronic disease focus too much on the next hospital visit, or a constant premonition that we are being picked on. "My intestines feel like they are attacking me," one of my clients told me.

Go away from your fears and move toward your desires. Many of us fear never-ending pain, hospitalization, even death. Yet, we desire digestive health and a more productive life for ourselves and families.

Ask yourself: What am I happy about in my life now? Who do I love? Who loves me? What am I grateful about?

Begin to see yourself in your mind's eye as being well, doing healthy things for yourself and others, and above all, constantly remind yourself of what *is* working well in your life. Many of the physically handicapped people I have worked with are remarkably optimistic. One should be thankful for the ability to see, hear, think, taste, dream, have a spouse, friends, family. Oftentimes we miss the small but precious things.

For healing to occur you must follow your heart. Those who overcome chronic disease have refused to be victims. When asked about his colon cancer, Ronald Reagan replied, "I didn't have cancer, I had something inside me that had cancer inside it, and it was removed."

Focus on Your Goals: Have a Mission in Life

One of the most important things a sick person can have is a personal mission. One of my favorite stories is of a friend whose wife was diagnosed with multiple sclerosis. While his wife watched others who were diagnosed at the same time become confined to wheelchairs, she had far fewer signs of her disease. Her secret? Her mission was to help kids at risk. Many of these children were placed temporarily into the couple's home while foster care arrangements were being made.

Quick Tips

- Make changes gradually
- Changes in weather, particularly cold and rainy weather, may make symptoms worse, therefore protect yourself from the elements as much as possible
- Walk after each meal
- Chew carefully (at least 7 times with each bite)
- Avoid tight-fitting garments, which can reduce the flow of blood

Why do some people live far longer than others? They have a mission. One of the healthiest 84-year-olds I know of is an herbalist who I practice with one day a week. He loves his work and there are so many people to help. He is simply too busy to fully retire. He worked a six-day week until he turned 80, then he began to work part-time.

Act "as if" you don't have a disorder. Ask yourself what you would like to contribute. What would you like to be doing? What do you love doing? I'll bet you could take small steps toward achieving your dreams. A mission does not have to be something you do full time or even what you do for a living, it's a way you can live your life.

Those who have overcome their conditions usually have a higher purpose to their lives that will not allow them to succumb to victimization by their disease. Healthy people cultivate positive emotions. Sick people cultivate negative emotions; they often don't have faith in getting better, they surround themselves with sick people, and they don't have a strong enough reason to get well.

You can either send the letter or simply keep it in your journal. Writing a letter to your digestive disorder is also good medicine. While emotions can also be explored with a counselor, therapist, or through a pastor, journaling is an unconventional technique that allows you to investigate hate, anger, or fear without feeling self-conscious. By writing your thoughts down, you can understand more fully some of the following issues: What is the worst possible outcome of your condition? What is the best possible outcome? What is the reason for your digestive disorder? Is it because of low self-esteem? Maybe you don't feel worthy of the life you are leading? Perhaps getting a flare-up is one way to avoid your present life. Or has stress become unbearable? How would you change this? Maybe you have never expressed, or are not aware of how others tried to control you? Is there anything your disease is trying to tell you?

Many of us feel like there is a volcano, a brick, a raw sore inhabiting our stomach and intestines. At one point during a horrific bout with Crohn's, I wondered if my stomach was inhabited by the devil. If I knew then what I know now, I would have coached myself to communicate with that feeling. One woman, Cassandra, named her aching gut Leo. "What are you up to now, Leo?" she would ask. "What are you trying to tell me?"

According to Jon Kabat-Zinn, PhD, associated with the University of Massachusetts Medical Center, paying attention to the pain and the various sensations of pain is more effective than trying to tune out the pain. This is because there are many pathways in the brain and the central nervous system that can modify the perception of pain. Dr. Kabat-Zinn is the author of the highly recommended book *Wherever You Go, There You Are.*[1]

Finally, keeping a journal is an excellent way to chart your progress. You can dedicate a page to writing down all your accomplishments and the peak experiences in your life. Read this page frequently throughout the day. This will mobilize your subconscious into helping heal your digestive system and reinforce the belief that you are worth healing.

Get Rid of the ANTs

Many of us have a constant barrage of thoughts, worries, and emotions that chatter endlessly at us. For those of us with chronic digestive disorders, at least part of that chatter is concerned with our stomach and intestines. For example, we may be bombarded with, *"When will my stomach stop bugging me . . . How am I going to give the talk at the 4-H Club tonight if my stomach doesn't stop . . . It feels like there's an aching, black hole down there . . . Maybe I should try meditating . . . No, it doesn't work . . . I wish I could get that raise so we can move . . . My wife says she's coming down with an ulcer, and my daughter doesn't want to go to school because of cramps . . . I wonder if I'll ever get that project in on time. . . ."*

No wonder many of us have chronic digestive disorders! By making an effort to reduce the negative chatter, we can allow ourselves to heal. For example, positive chatter might be, *"I'm glad I have a wife and three kids . . . Maybe I do feel better after drinking all that peppermint tea . . . I'm sure I'll get the raise . . . What's the worst thing that can happen to me at the 4-H Club—I'll make a fool out of myself in front of some fourth graders!? . . . I wonder if I should go see that acupuncturist for my pain . . . It worked for James; it changed his life."* It is important to fill both one's conscious and subconscious mind with positive self-talk.

One of my clients, Carl, told me, "I always worry. My life should be perfect. I just got married, my career is going well, I don't even work very hard, yet I'm constantly worrying!" My advice was to get the ANTs out of his head. ANTs stands for **A**utomatic **N**egative **T**houghts. Your head is filled with old "tapes," inserted by people in your past. They may be your par-

Begin an Exercise
and Stress Reduction Program

The backbone of healing your digestive system is a commitment to one hour of exercise every day, or a combination of exercise and stress reduction (meditation, prayer, tai chi, yoga). I have seen people who make and follow through with this commitment get better; those who cannot make this commitment often do not make lasting improvement.

When we exercise, our blood flow is increased. When our blood flow is increased, oxygen is delivered more rapidly and effectively to our body tissues. Oxygen to the brain helps sharpen alertness as well as reduce anxiety and depression. Modern research has found that exercise assists the body in creating natural chemicals called endorphins, which help to elevate our mood. Exercise also promotes sound sleep, because everything is running more efficiently. Exercise tones all our muscles, including those of the bowel, thus elimination is regulated.

To me, exercise means a pleasant activity done vigorously enough so that one does not spend time thinking about one's problems. If possible, find a friend you can exercise with in order to give each other mutual support. The exercise you choose should be one that works for you, that is, it brings you the most amount of enjoyment. What sports do you enjoy? Aerobics, biking, rowing, jogging, hiking, racquet sports, or ball games? Group exercises such as aerobics or team sports are fast-paced, so that you do not have time to worry about your personal problems. Stationary bicycles, step and rowing machines, and equipment that simulates cross country skiing are also beneficial. Swimming is said to be one of the best exercises, because it puts the least amount of strain on the joints while giving you an all-around workout.

If you are not in good shape, vigorous walking will do. For several reasons, walking in the country or in a park is better than walking in the city or in a shopping mall. Exposure to nature is very important to the healing process, whereas city walking exposes one to pollution as well as other discordant distractions. When walking in nature, notice how your body feels touching the ground. Notice the flowers and animals. Notice the trees and grass. If there is a pond, notice what is being reflected.

There is no doubt that the first thirty days of making this commitment are the hardest. But you must bear in mind your goal of getting healthy and of your mission in life. If necessary, get up an hour earlier. Most people find that after thirty days of daily relaxation and exercise, it is their favorite part of the day, and is frequently the only time for solitude. Some parents with toddlers buy a sports stroller with bicycle-like tires to either run or speed walk with their young ones. And when their children are older, they strap them into a child's seat on a bike. Aside from the obvious immediate benefits, youngsters are exposed to the importance of exercise at an early age, hopefully preparing them to continue with activity throughout their lives.

Quick Tips for Relieving Digestive Symptoms

- Rub your belly in a clockwise direction 100 times every day
- To relieve gas, hold your knees in front of your chest while lying on the floor
- Practice good posture
- Warmth such as heating pads or warm baths may be useful
- Take a hot shower until your stomach turns red (allow the water to directly spray the stomach). Be careful not to burn yourself!

At the other end of the age spectrum, many of the healthiest seniors follow a program of good diet and exercise, which is why they live to such advanced ages. At the YMCA I belong to, there are many senior activities, including aerobics and swimming, as well as outings.

The only people who shouldn't follow this program are those

Take a Hot Bath

One of the most powerful weapons against digestive disorders is the most gentle: a hot bath or sauna. Heat helps relax muscles and joints. Heat also releases stress hormones, which make it less likely that we overreact to stress. Ideally the bath should be as hot as one can stand it. Continually add hot water as necessary. Essential oils of lavender can be added. Also, herbs such as chamomile and lemon balm may be brewed as tea and added to the bath (see this chapter for directions). Some people find that a heating pad or a hot water bottle applied to the stomach and intestines works better than a bath.

Get a Massage

You can buy a portable massager, use your own hands, or pay a masseuse. The best alternative is a spouse or friend. My suggestion is to begin with the feet, and end at the head, spending plenty of time with your stomach (see abdominal self-massage, Chapter Four) spine, shoulders, neck, and forehead. Mechanical self-massagers help get you to these areas. Pressure may be also applied to tender points in the body, ears, hands, and feet to ease digestive and other symptoms.

Make Time for Hobbies

Distress causes your head to become gray; anger speeds aging; laughter makes you ten years younger. —Chinese proverb

How many people work long hours and then park themselves in front of the TV? How many hours each day do you spend reading the newspaper or watching the news? Chatting on

Stress Reducing Bath Number 1

Once the bath has been drawn, add 5 drops of marjoram, 5 drops of lavender, 5 drops of chamomile. Epsom salts may be added after as well, following directions on the label. Cover up after your bath and listen to a stress reduction tape.

Stress Reducing Bath Number 2

Make a strong brew of chamomile and lemon balm tea, strain, and pour into the bath.

Digestive Bath

While drawing the bath, add 1 teaspoon of peppermint oil, or place 2 peppermint tea bags into the tub; add Epsom salts once the bath is drawn.

Warming Bath

Pour 1 to 3 teaspoons of powdered ginger into the bath water. If you have sensitive skin, use fresh ginger by putting a 2 inch slice in an old sock or muslin bag. You can also add 5 cinnamon sticks. You should break out into a sweat. It is important to dry off well, cover up in a blanket as soon as you get out of the bath.

the phone? Window-shopping? None of these activities enrich your life. Once, I read about a Buddhist monk who advised his American students to give up meditation, and just spend thirty minutes a day laughing. If you must watch movies, watch comedies!

Many of us have forgotten simple pleasures that give the mind a rest, such as hiking, walking, crafts, playing a musical instrument, or participating in hobbies. Success, even in small things, supports a feeling of self-confidence and self-worth.

breakfast is the most important meal of the day. If we establish regular times for meals and eat "like a king for breakfast, a prince for lunch, and a pauper for dinner," we are well on our way to good health. Too many Americans eat next to nothing for breakfast, eat lunch on the run, then sit down for a big dinner late at night. No wonder our digestive systems are in an uproar!

Generally, people with digestive problems do better eating four to six small meals throughout the day, rather that two or three large meals. Eating too much at one sitting overburdens the digestive process. Constant snacking, or eating late at night, also does not give your digestive system a chance to rest. Make a habit of eating until only three fourths full—stop *before* you are stuffed.

Before eating say a prayer of thanks. Ask yourself if you really want to eat the food in front of you. If you are tense or nervous, wait until the tension has passed. If the food is unappealing, select something that will nourish your body. Ask yourself what you really want to eat. "Is this what my body really wants?" The answer may surprise you. Your body might do better with protein and vegetables for breakfast, and oatmeal at dinner.

Observe the colors and the texture of the food in front of you. Who was involved in producing it? Smell your food. In order to slow down your eating, use chopsticks. Slow, soothing music may help slow down the speed at which you eat.

Chew your food well. Savor each bite. In some parts of the world they recommend chewing each bite of food fifty times before swallowing. I usually advise my American clients to deliberately chew at least seven times. This makes good sense, as chewing allows digestive enzymes from the salivary glands to mix with food. Eating slowly prevents swallowing air, so that bloating is avoided. I have observed people in fast food restaurants: They don't even chew—they just bite and wash down the food with a gulp of carbonated beverage. Not only can carbonated beverages cause irritation to the stomach, but excessive amounts of liquids consumed with meals dilute digestive enzymes: bloating is the result.

Make mealtimes as relaxing as possible. Meals take several hours in many parts of the world. When you eat, just eat. Do not watch television, argue, or conduct business. Make a contest to see how slowly you can eat. One client found his IBS cured after a visit to Greece, where meals are eaten at a snail's pace, and home-made yogurt is served with each meal. After eating, don't go back to work or engage in any rigorous physical activity right away. Go for a walk. The Chinese say: "Walk one hundred paces after meals and one can live ninety-nine years."

Eat Foods Warm

For centuries, the Chinese have adhered to the custom of eating most foods cooked

Check Your Thyroid

Thyroid imbalance may be causing your digestive symptoms

According to some holistic doctors, constipation, bloating, poor appetite, and digestion may be caused by hypothyroidism (low thyroid hormone levels). Hyperthyroidism (excess thyroid hormone levels) may cause diarrhea or loose bowel movements, weight loss, and other symptoms, such as palpitations, anxiety, insomnia, and goiter.

and warm, as opposed to raw and cold. Cooked food, according to the Chinese, requires less energy to turn into fuel. Warm food benefits the stomach and entire digestive system by helping to maintain the flow of energy. Cold food causes the energy to slow down and even become "stuck," resulting in digestive problems. American patients who habitually drink ice cold beverages, eat cold sandwiches, salads, and iced desserts, would do well to follow this Chinese custom. Individuals with digestive disorders should eat everything cooked and warm, or at least at room temperature. Eating according to season is also important. Therefore,

Eat Healing Foods

There is no such thing as a "best" diet. If you have a digestive disorder, you are probably more sensitive to food than most people. Although there are some foods that seem to react with a large number of people, they do not react with everyone. Therefore it is important that you pay attention to your body and become familiar with its likes and dislikes.

Most people make two common mistakes. First, they force themselves to eat foods they assume are good for them. Second, they ignore reactions to food cravings. Later in this chapter, there is a food sensitivity list of foods likely to cause digestive symptoms. An example of the former is salads. Americans universally assume that salads are good for them. In terms of Chinese medicine, salads are cold in property and should not be eaten by people with weak digestive systems. This is particularly true during the winter months, when the weather may have adverse consequences on one's health. Salads are also contraindicated in terms of Western medicine during gastrointestinal flare-ups, as they contain roughage. In practical terms this means that some individuals can never eat salads and must have all vegetables cooked. Some can eat salads in the summer but not in winter, and others can eat salads only with the help of the herbal and dietary supplements mentioned in this book. Still others find that warming spices such as black pepper and fennel are helpful in offsetting the cold property of salads.

In terms of protein, getting an adequate amount is important. Protein is made up of amino acids, which are the building blocks of life. All body tissues, functions, and processes involve proteins. The best protein sources are animal products such as meat and fish. Try eating small amounts of meat or fish with every meal. In many Asian countries, meat is often stir-fried with vegetables. In this way, the flavoring and protein of meat are combined with the health benefit of vegetables. Many people with chronic digestive disorders are intolerant of excess fat, and should therefore eat only lean meat.

Fats

Following a lowfat diet is important if you have a chronic digestive disorder. You may have already found this out. Fats are more likely to cause diarrhea, gas, bloating, and belching than other foods. However, not all fats are to be avoided. Try to use oils like olive or canola (unsaturated fat) that are liquid, rather than butter (saturated fat), which is solid at room temperature.

Studies conducted in Denmark and Japan indicate that persons whose diets contain both Omega 3 and Omega 6 oils have a much lower incidence of inflammatory disease. Omega 6 oils are found in corn, sunflower, and soy oils, as well as in animal fat. In order to increase our ratio of Omega 3 oils, we can eat more fish, avocados, flax, canola, rapeseed, and sesame seed oils, or take supplemental EPA. The following fish contain Omega 3 oils: salmon, mackerel, anchovy, cod, striped bass, snapper, haddock, sardine, trout, and tuna.

Banana

According to a medical study conducted in India, 75 percent of patients who took banana powder capsules experienced complete or partial relief from dyspepsia.[6] Bananas also help build a strong barrier between the stomach lining and gastric acid, thus protecting against ulcers.

Cabbage

Cabbage strengthens the stomach lining and protects against ulcers. A study conducted by Garrett Cheney, MD, professor of medicine

Eliminate Smoking, Alcohol, and Sweets

The alcoholic, the cigarette or marijuana smoker, and the modern office worker who must eat chocolate or other sweets have more in common than you may think. All of these habits contribute to low blood sugar, medically known as hypoglycemia. Hypoglycemia can cause many digestive symptoms such as constant hunger, craving for sweets, gastrointestinal pain, food cravings, and indigestion, in addition to fatigue, depression, irritability, and headaches. According to some nutritionists, it is possible to have symptoms of low blood sugar even though all medical tests are normal. In his book *Low Blood Sugar,*[7] Dr. Martin Budd states: "I find that many patients suffering from stomach ulcers, heartburn, hiatal hernia, and other digestive ailments often have a blood sugar imbalance." Low blood sugar can be corrected by the following measures:

- Avoid sugar, sweets, and artificial sweeteners
- Eliminate alcohol, smoking, and recreational drugs
- Eat protein in the morning
- Use protein or whole fruits to counter sweet cravings
- Eat four to six light meals per day

Identify Food Triggers

The following is a list of foods that are widely known to trigger digestive symptoms. They are not all unhealthy foods. You may find after eliminating one or more of these foods that your digestive symptoms are reduced. It is important to go at least one week (preferably two weeks) without a food to determine whether or not it is the cause of the symptoms.

Preservatives, flavorings, processing aids, nutritional additives, and even cookware may also trigger digestive symptoms. Therefore, your diet should emphasize fresh foods whenever possible. A complete digestive clearing plan is discussed in Chapter Five.

Milk and Dairy Products

Milk can lead to a broad spectrum of complaints and is probably the greatest cause of food intolerance. Milk can give rise to intestinal gas, diarrhea, heartburn, dyspepsia, stomatitis, gallbladder attacks, pancreatitis, IBD flare-ups, duodenal ulcer, and hemorrhoids. Other manifestations of milk intolerance are asthma, bedwetting, migraine, and hayfever. It is the constant use of milk and other dairy products, especially in childhood, that gradually weakens the digestive system and leads to the abovementioned symptoms.

Milk contains lactose. Under normal circumstances, lactose is broken down into glucose and galactose by the enzyme lactase. If the body is unable to digest and absorb lactose, it remains in the intestines, where it interferes with normal intestinal bacteria, thus leading to cramps, gas, bloating, and diarrhea. Lactose intolerance is more common among older people and in non-northern Europeans. You can experiment with lactase drops or supplements. Some milk already has lactate in it. I am one of the many people who is not lactose intolerant according to medical tests, but who cannot tolerate milk. In fact, humans are the only animals who as adults drink milk! Some people are able to tolerate goat but not cow milk. Dairy products include milk, butter, cream, butterfat, powdered or condensed milk, whey, yogurt, cheese, ice cream, casein (a component of milk also referred to as caseinate), lactose, lactate, nonfat milk solids or lactalbumin (another component of milk).

Sweets, Sugars, and Artificial Sweeteners

All sweets including artificial sweeteners can cause digestive symptoms. Chocolate can give rise to immediate reactions such as

Asian Restaurant Syndrome

The problem with the Asian diet for non-Asians is that it contains soy products such as teriyaki and soy sauce, which many Americans are allergic to. The Asian diet also consists of many fermented foods, which are contraindicated for those who have candida complex. A further problem is MSG (monosodium glutamate), which can lead to upset stomach, thirst, dizziness, headaches, tiredness, high blood pressure, and rashes.

Soy

Many persons have intolerance to soybeans and other soy products such as tofu and soy sauce. Restaurants, especially fast food chains, cook with soy oil or flour. Soy flour is also used by bakers in breads, cakes, rolls, and pastries. Some crackers contain soybean flour. Salad dressings often contain soybean oil.

Wheat

Wheat sensitivity is known to cause dyspepsia, heartburn, and diarrhea, as well as migraine, fatigue, emotional upset, and dermatitis herpetiformis. The component of wheat that induces the sensitivity is gluten. Gluten intolerance is known as celiac disease. Other gluten-containing foods include rye, oat, and barley.

Corn

Corn is difficult to avoid as it is ubiquitous in manufactured foods. Some patients are able to tolerate fresh corn off the cob, but not canned corn or other forms of corn and cornmeal. While corn can cause acute reactions, it is more likely to gradually weaken the digestive system, leading to symptoms such as gastritis, colitis, allergic rhinitis (hayfever), asthma, migraine and hives. Corn is found in Mexican food and chips, and in alcoholic beverages including beer, ale, brandy, gin, whiskey, and vodka. It may be contained in wines, including the sparkling variety. Dextrose is corn sugar and glucose is corn syrup. Corn is found in talcum powder, bath oils and powders, and clothing starch.

Nuts

Nuts are high in fat and cause allergic reactions in millions of Americans. Peanuts and peanut butter are a frequent cause of dyspepsia and migraine.

Yeast and Fermented Foods

Yeast is commonly used in food preparation. It converts sugars to alcohol and carbon dioxide in a fermentation process. Yeast and mold may lead to a cross-reactivity in some hypersensitive people. Sauerkraut, vinegar, and miso may aggravate digestive symptoms.

Eggs

Eggs can give rise to gallbladder flare-ups, gastritis, dyspepsia, migraine, asthma, diarrhea, acne, and hives. Eggs are often contaminated with salmonella, which can cause a host of digestive disorders and even sore joints. Powdered eggs are of particular risk for salmonella. Therefore, egg dishes must be heated thoroughly to 106°F (41°C). In addition, *do not eat raw eggs!* Eggs may also contain pesticide residues, antibiotics, and hormones. Some individuals are only allergic to the egg white, not the yolk. Albumin, levetin, ovomucin, ovomucoid, and vitellin indicate the presence of eggs or egg components. For persons sensitive to chicken eggs, duck, goose, turkey, ostrich, or turtle eggs may be substituted.

Healthcare Issues
Create a Healthcare Team

Chronic disease can make you feel powerless; taking control of your health can help you feel empowered. Select health professionals who have empathy as well as skill. It may not be realistic to expect to find a compassionate doctor who is also the most up-to-date on the latest research. Choose the balance that feels the most comfortable to you.

Most medical doctors are not aware of the breadth of natural medicine. One of my clients, after having experienced great results at our clinic, wondered why his medical doctor had never told him about the benefits of herbs. I explained that if you want a diagnosis and treatment based on Western medicine, you go to a Western medical doctor. If you want herbs for your condition, you must go to an herbalist. Whether you see a medical doctor or a holistic practitioner, here are some suggestions:

- Write down a list of questions before meeting with your health professional. Let him/her know at the beginning of the meeting that you have questions. Inquire about costs, treatment and diagnostic options, risks and side effects associated with drugs and surgery. What is the length of time you should expect before you see results? What are the possible consequences of delaying medication or surgery in order to try natural healing methods? Can surgery or toxic drugs (such as chemotherapy) be scheduled after, rather than before, your vacation?
- Don't hide your symptoms. Although you may be embarrassed to talk about your bowel movements, or abdominal pain, it is important to be as specific as possible. *All too often patients wait until the end of the visit to convey the most important information.*

- If you are meeting with a holistic health professional, explain when your symptoms began, and state what you think the cause is. If you have any unhealthy habits that could be contributing to your health problem, it is crucial that you bring these up, as your practitioner may have helpful suggestions.
- If possible, bring a spouse or a friend with you. Companions can help reduce your anxiety in the waiting room, help you remember to ask certain questions during your appointment, and can accompany you to a meal or favorite activity afterward.

Health professionals are human. If they do something you don't like, share your feelings. It is always more productive to make "I feel" statements rather than statements such as: "You did this . . . , you don't care about me." If you are unable to speak up, consider writing a letter to your health professional.

In addition to your medical doctor, you may want to incorporate a specialist in one of the following areas. Ask a friend or colleague for a referral, or you may write to me (see Resource Guide) for a health professional who practices herbology.

- **Herbalist:** Look for one who practices full time or who has another specialty, such as acupuncture. Feel free to ask about his/her training; the usual training consists of either formal academic training or apprenticeship. It has been my experience that properly recommended herbs can make a great difference in digestive health. An herbalist should offer dietary and lifestyle counseling, and may or may not be knowledgeable about dietary supplements.
- **Nutritional Counselor:** Herbalists, nutritionists, acupuncturists, and medical doctors practice nutritional counseling. A nutritionist can offer suggestions about diet as well as lifestyle changes, and recommend specific dietary supplements. Dietitians are knowledgeable about meal plans, but they are usually not healers.

49

Under the guidance of an herbalist or another holistic health professional, herbal formulas can be administered to rid the body of unhealthy pathogens. Probiotic supplements, such as acidophilus and bifidus, can be used to introduce healthy bacteria into your gut; and fructooligosaccharides (FOS) and colostrom to help normalize your GI system. Specific dietary supplements can correct nutrient deficiencies, and herbal and vegetable enzymes can be used to help food assimilate more easily (see the "Candidiasis" and "Parasites" sections in Chapter Four).

Stay Informed about Surgery and Pharmaceutical Medications

Question all medical procedures, and if possible, read up about them. In some cases, such as barium enemas, the risks may outweigh the benefits. Surgery does not guarantee that you will be without symptoms. Countless people undergo operations that only temporarily relieve their problems. Many surgeries are not medically necessary. Make an informed decision by doing your own research. Information is available through libraries as well as online. Whenever possible, get a second opinion before undergoing any surgery for a chronic illness.

Make a list of any medications you are taking. Look these up in the *Physician's Desk Reference (PDR)* or *Nurse's Drug Guide,* available at a public library or bookstore. Find out if any of these medications have digestive side effects. Meet with your physician, pharmacist, and holistic health professional to find out if there are alternatives to these medications that won't upset your digestion. Before starting on any drugs, you should know about their risks. The following are categories of medications that are known to have digestion-related side effects.

Antibiotics

While no one denies that antibiotics are one of the greatest medical discoveries of all time, their overuse and misuse are currently a serious health problem. In fact, at a recent Congressional hearing, evidence was presented that an estimated 40 to 60 percent of prescriptions for antibiotics in America are incorrect.

Antibiotics are not only over-administered to humans, but they are used as growth enhancers and for disease prevention in the raising of chickens, turkeys, pigs, and cattle. There are several problems with the overuse of antibiotics. First, bacteria can develop a resistance to antibiotics, because they are able to change their chemistry and genes in such a way that the antibiotics have little or no effect. This process is speeded up when you do not finish your antibiotic prescriptions. Second, antibiotics kill off not only the bad bacteria, but also the good bacteria necessary to protect us from opportunistic infections. Good bacteria help to crowd out invading bacteria by attaching to the intestinal wall, thus preventing the invading bacteria and fungus from reducing the integrity of the intestinal tract. If all the good bacteria are killed off, the bad bacteria can take over. If you have ants in your house, leave food out, and do not clean, pretty soon the ants will take over your house.

By misuse we are talking about antibiotics being misprescribed. In other words, antibiotics are prescribed for the wrong conditions, or for diseases for which their use is not warranted. A case in point are viral conditions—you should never insist that your doctor prescribe antibiotics for viral infections, as these medications are ineffective for such conditions.

Antacids

Antacids are used to suppress stomach acid. The aluminum in these products can cause constipation. Adults with metabolic bone diseases should not take them, nor should they be used for prolonged periods by those with kidney diseases. Holistic doctors caution the use of aluminum products, as they may contribute to Alzheimer's disease. Do not take antacids for longer than two weeks without consulting with your health professional.

Anti-Nausea Drugs

Compazine (prochlorperazine), Tigan (trimethobenzamide), and Antivert (Meclizine) are used to treat motion sickness. These medications may cause confusion, delirium, short-term memory problems, disorientation, dry mouth, constipation, difficulty urinating, blurred vision, and worsening of glaucoma. There are many interactions with other drugs, which you should review with your pharmacist.

Sulfazine (Azulfidine, Asacol, Rowasa)

Sulfazine is used to treat Crohn's disease and ulcerative colitis. Sulfazine depletes the body of folic acid, making supplementation necessary. Adverse effects include itching, aching joints or muscles, difficulty swallowing, fever, sore throat, abnormal bleeding or bruising, weakness or tiredness, and yellow eyes and skin. Complete blood counts, proctoscopy, sigmoidoscopy, urine tests, and liver and kidney function tests should be administered if you take sulfazine over long periods.

Ulcer Drugs (Tagomet, Zantac, Pepcid, Axid, Prilosec, Prevacid, Cytotec)

These drugs should not be taken for minor digestive complaints such as occasional upset stomach, nausea, or heartburn, as they suppress stomach acid. Stomach acid helps destroy viruses, fungi, and unwanted bacteria, and aids in the absorption of nutrients. The above reasons explain why many who take these drugs have a relapse within two years of starting on them.

Adverse effects include confusion, hallucinations, sore throat and fever, unusual bleeding or bruising, irregular heartbeat, and unusual tiredness or weakness. Call your health professional if you have decreased sexual functioning, diarrhea, dizziness or headache, muscle cramps or pain, skin rash, or enlarged or sore breasts. If you have reduced liver or kidney function, you need to decrease the dosages of these drugs.

Prilosec and Prevacid treat conditions that don't respond to usual acid blockers or antacids. In laboratory experiments, Prilosec caused an increase in stomach tumors, therefore it is not recommended for long-term therapy, except for the treatment of ZE, a very rare disease. Side effects, which may require immediate medical attention, include bleeding or bruising, difficulty breathing, fever, mouth sores, sore throat, fatigue, and cloudy or bloody urine. If you continue to have gastrointestinal symptoms, anxiety or depression, bodily aches and pains, skin reactions, respiratory difficulties, or painful erections or breast enlargement in men, consult your health professional or pharmacist.

Cytotec (misoprostol) is used to prevent ulcers caused by NSAIDS such as aspirin and ibuprofen. Those who have had Crohn's or ulcerative colitis should not use it. The common side effects include diarrhea, abdominal pain, flatulence, and headache.

Corticosteroids (Prednisone)

Corticosteroids, such as prednisone, are used to treat Crohn's disease and ulcerative colitis; they suppress the immune system. If you take corticosteroids over long periods, your risk of infection as well as of osteoporosis are increased. There are many possible side effects from long-term use, such as abdominal pain, skin problems, moon face, increased blood pressure, weight gain, irregular heartbeat, muscle cramps, fatigue, bodily pain or weakness, nausea and vomiting, thin skin, bruising easily, wounds that will not heal, eye disorders, euphoria, depression, trouble sleeping, nosebleeds, increased facial or body hair, insomnia, facial flushing, and anxiety. When on corticosteroids, regular eye exams should be undertaken, and glucose concentration, hypothalamus and pituitary functions, and blood loss should all be monitored. Potassium, sodium, and calcium levels should also be evaluated. Reducing corticosteroids should be done gradually, under the supervision of your health professional.

Drugs for Excess Gas

According the editors of *Worst Pills Best Pills,*[9] anti-gas formulas containing simethicone are a waste of money, as there is no convincing evidence that they are effective. (See "Intestinal Gas" section, Chapter Four, for more effective treatments.)

Anti-Diarrhea Drugs

Medications such as Lomotil and Motofen treat severe diarrhea. Long-term use can cause many mental and physical side effects. Imodium A-D is more innocuous in that its side effects are minimal. Anti-diarrhea drugs should never be taken in excess of the recommended dosage. They are also habit-forming, thus long-term usage should be avoided. These drugs must be used carefully—if at all—for infectious diarrhea, as they may delay recovery by slowing down the removal of toxic bacteria or viruses, or of parasites. Diarrhea that does not respond to these drugs may indicate an infection due to these pathogens.

Relaxants (Used for IBS, Ulcers, Colitis, Crohn's Disease)

Relaxants that have antispasmodic properties treat cramping associated with the above disorders. These drugs can cause confusion, memory problems and disorientation, dry mouth, sexual dysfunction, difficulty urinating and worsening of glaucoma. Relaxants should never be stopped suddenly, but should be tapered off under the supervision of your health professional. If possible, use herbal relaxants, take hot baths, and apply topical essential oils.

Psyllium Products

Psyllium is an herb that is found in many preparations in health food stores and pharmacies; it is used to help move the intestines. It is far better to eat a high fiber diet and drink plenty of liquids than to rely on psyllium products, as these often contain excess sugar. If raw vegetables seem to be irritating, try cooking or pureeing your vegetables. Some people have better results with more soluble fibers, such as oat bran and guar gum. Take medications at least an hour apart from psyllium products, because the latter may interfere with absorption of pharmaceuticals.

Laxatives

Long-term use of laxatives is habit-forming. If you have become dependent on laxatives, seek the help of your health professional. Some chemical laxatives have serious side effects, such as danthron, a cancer-causing agent, which was recalled in the United

States. Docusate, a stool softener, among other laxatives, can cause irreparable intestinal damage as well as interfere with the body's absorption of nutrients and other drugs. Some laxatives contain excessive amounts of sugar, salt, and/or artificial sweeteners.

Nicotine

Anecdotal evidence indicates that some individuals who stop smoking develop colitis. It could be that nicotine alleviates some of the symptoms associated with ulcerative colitis. In a study published in the *New England Journal of Medicine,* patients using nicotine patches had less abdominal pain and decreased stool frequency and urgency than a group that was placed on placebo patches (patches that did not contain any medicine at all).[10] However, there were more side effects for those on the nicotine patches as opposed to the subjects on placebo patches. If all other techniques fail, nicotine patches may be a possible therapy to be used along with standard care for ulcerative colitis. However, smokers should quit smoking anyway, as it is associated with other health risks such as cancer.

Cancer Drugs

Chemotherapy drugs often cause severe nausea and vomiting. Before trying anti-nausea drugs, try eating small meals throughout the day so that your stomach is not empty. Snacks such as crackers or toast, as well as clear liquids, are helpful, as are tart foods such as lemons and pickles. Digestive Harmony (Quiet Digestion) is an herbal formula that has helped many people who suffer from the side effects of chemotherapy drugs.

Chapter Notes

1. Jon Kabat-Zinn, *Wherever You Go, There You Are* (New York, NY: St. Martin's Press, 1994).

2. Louise Hay, *You Can Heal Your Life* (Carson, CA: Hay House, 1989.

3. David Burns, *The Feeling Good Handbook* (New York, NY: Penguin Books, 1989).

4. F. Batmanghelidj, "A New and Natural Method of Treatment of Peptic Ulcer Disease," *Journal of Clinical Gastroenterology* 5 (1983) 203-205.

5. F. Batmanghelidj, *Your Body's Many Cries for Water* (Falls Church, VA: Global Health Solutions).

6. Jean Carper, *Food: Your Miracle Medicine* (New York: HarperCollins, 1993) 133.

7. Martin Budd, *Low Blood Sugar* (New York, NY: Sterling Publishing, 1981).

8. J.C. Brenenman, *Basics of Food Allergy* (Springfield, IL: Charles C Thomas, 1978).

9. Sidney Wolfe, *Worst Pills, Best Pills* (Washington, DC: Public Citizen's Health Research Group, 1993).

10. R.D. Pullan, J. Rhodes, S. Ganesh, V. Mani, J.S. Morris, G.T. Williams, R.G. Newcombe, M.A. Russell, C. Feyerabend, G.A. Thomas, et al., "Transdermal Nicotine for Active Ulcerative Colitis," *New England Journal of Medicine* 330 (1994) 811.

Chapter Three

Natural Therapies

This chapter discusses effective therapies to heal your digestive system. These remedies can be used with any medication you are taking. It is advisable to take these supplements under the guidance of a knowledgeable health professional, who can select the most effective remedies for your signs and symptoms. Many people who attempt self-treatment do not take the correct products or the correct dosages. The best way to find a professional with experience using natural therapies is by word of mouth. Also, if you write to me, I may be able to locate a practitioner in your area (see Resource Guide at end of this book).

Under the guidance of a professional, you should expect to see some improvement within the first thirty days, however it may take six months or longer for a drastic reduction in your symptoms to occur. If you do not feel at least somewhat better in your overall energy level after thirty days, bring this to the attention of your professional. If he or she is unable to adjust your protocol and provide you some relief, request a referral.

When beginning natural therapies it is possible, though not likely, to have what is known as a healing crisis. The most common symptoms are a worsening in digestive symptoms, skin rashes, or discharges. I recommend starting herbs and dietary supplements at a reduced dosage to avoid these reactions.

Whereas vitamin and mineral preparations are used to treat specific deficiencies and to help improve one's nutritional status, herbal medicines, when properly combined, can manage many digestive symptoms with far fewer side effects than Western drugs.

It should be pointed out that these remedies are considered dietary supplements, not medications, and are not researched in the way that drugs are. Information about these formulas has been gathered on the basis of historical usage, which includes a great deal of trial and error. Finally, never discontinue prescribed medications without consulting your physician.

Digestive Herbs

Herbology is an energetic medicine. Plants have a life force: the Chinese call it "Qi" (pronounced "chee"). Imagine being in an office building all day, staring at a computer and dealing with fax machines and telephones, without a window nearby to view the outside. Now, think about a day when you were outside in nature walking along and viewing peaceful scenery with the sunlight on your face. Which feels better to you? By taking herbs we are bringing the life force of nature inside our bodies.

The therapeutic action of herbs is not as pronounced as pharmaceutical medications, meaning that herbs have fewer side effects and are more easily tolerated. Herbs may be taken in tincture, tea, tablet, or powder form. Generally, those with digestive disorders should not take alcohol tinctures as the alcohol may be too warming and may spread pathogenic yeast. Furthermore,

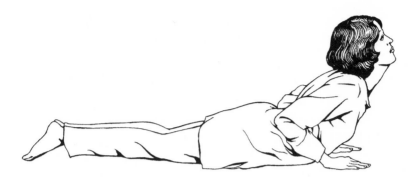

Cobra

The cobra position improves circulation and helps relieve intestinal gas pain, cramps, and backache. Lie on your stomach with the your forehead resting on the floor. Your legs and feet should be extended while your body is relaxed. Place your hands palms down next to your chest, keeping your fingertips aligned with your breasts. While inhaling, slowly raise your head, then your shoulders and finally chest, without using your arms or hands. Look upward and extend back as far as possible. Hold for 5 seconds. Exhale. Lower your body until your forehead again rests on the floor. Relax. Repeat this exercise at least 20 times.

Tip: Your navel should remain on the floor during this exercise. Use the muscles of your back to push your body off the floor, not your arms and legs. **You should experience stretching in the waist and neck, not straining or pain.**

---

alcohol is an inefficient way to consume herbs. Teas, tablets, and powders allow you to take in a much higher dosage of herbs. In addition to addressing specific digestive disorders, herbs may be taken for stress and tension, as well as for colds and the flu.

In terms of when herbs should be taken, in general they are more efficiently absorbed on an empty stomach. Most tablet and capsule products should be taken with a large glass of hot or room-temperature water, or with hot herbal tea when called for. Herbal teas may also be taken immediately before meals. Some formulas such as Digestive Harmony (Quiet Digestion) are administered before, during, or after meals in order to help food digest and assimilate.

Whereas some herbs such as peppermint tea belong in every digestive patient's kitchen, others, particularly Chinese herbs, should be administered under the guidance of a trained professional. The remainder of this chapter discusses which natural products can be self-administered, which should be taken with caution, and which should be taken only under the guidance of a qualified practitioner.

Herbs That Can Be Self-Administered

Flower Essences

Flower essences are liquid extracts that are used to address mind-body health. The English physician, Dr. Edward Bach, did important research on the application of flower essences for specific emotions. Although he was conventionally trained, he based his treatments on emotions rather than on physical diagnosis. He was able to correlate specific wild flowers with states of mind. Flower essences are not used to treat specific disease, but may be particularly useful in addressing stress and depression associated with digestive and other disorders. Flower essences are produced differently than regular herbal products, using only the fresh blossoms of the plant, which are prepared by infusion. For example, dill, when used traditionally, stimulates digestion and treats intestinal gas. As a flower essence, dill is used when the soul feels overwhelmed.

Flower essences can be combined with other healing modalities. They are particularly beneficial for persons who are sensitive and for those who are not able to tolerate regular herb products. The Rescue Remedy, also known as the Five Flower Remedy, is widely available in health food stores and is useful to take before, after, and during stressful or traumatic events.

Aromatherapy (Essential Oils)

Essential oils are fragrant substances derived from plants. They are packaged in liquid form to be used topically, in baths, or in a diffuser to allow the fragrance to permeate an entire room. They are not meant for internal use unless specified by your herbal supplier. Essential oils are especially good as adjuncts to internal herbs, or for individuals who are hypersensitive and unable to tolerate internal herbs. Eucalyptus is an example: It

How to Make Herbal Tea

Glass or ceramic pots make the best tea.

- **Dried, Cut, and Sifted Herbs:** Flowers, leaves, and thin stems are steeped with the lid on for 10 to 15 minutes. Use 1 cup of boiling water to 1 teaspoon of powdered or 1 tablespoon of lighter dried herbs (e.g., flowers) per cup. Strain before drinking the tea.
- **Dried, Whole Herbs:** roots, bark, and heavy stems should be simmered for 20 minutes. For whole herbs, use about 1 oz (30 g) of herbs per 16 oz of boiling water. Strain before drinking.
- **Chinese Herbs:** Prepare by boiling for longer periods of time as directed by your herbalist.
- **Herbs in Tea Bags:** Steep in a teapot or cup with the lid on for 5 to 10 minutes.

is widely used as a steam therapy for bronchial and nasal conditions, as well as in over-the-counter chest rub for colds.

Fragrant smells or subtle changes in odor affect the central nervous system. Some essential oils are considered stimulants, while others are relaxants. In the treatment of digestive disorders they are used either to relax the gastrointestinal tract or to stimulate peristalsis. For example, 40 drops of peppermint or chamomile oil can be combined with 3 ounces of almond oil, olive oil, or water. Knead into the entire stomach and intestinal area by rubbing clockwise. Another essential oil, lavender, taken alone or with other herbs, can be applied topically to the skin during times of stress. I find an anti-stress blend of chamomile, marjoram, laudanum, lavender, and orange to be very soothing before public speaking. I place a drop on the inside of my wrists, to the back of my neck, and behind my ears.

Peppermint

I consider peppermint the queen of digestive herbs. The best peppermint for this purpose is fresh domestic peppermint. Other mints such as spearmint have similar though milder effects. Peppermint is available in tea bags or as a loose tea. Peppermint oil can also be used. Generally peppermint tea is more soothing, particularly to the digestive system, whereas peppermint oil is more stimulating. Since the active constituents of peppermint are fragile, don't boil the herb, instead let it steep with a lid on the teapot.

For gastric acidity, indigestion, or digestive related headache, apply peppermint oil drops directly on the temples, between the eyebrows, on the forehead, back of the neck, or behind the ears. Drops may also be placed on the abdomen over the liver, stomach, and intestines; massage in a clockwise motion. For intestinal spasm use peppermint oil externally, and drink a warm cup of peppermint tea. For nausea or dry heaves, sip 2 drops of peppermint oil placed in a half cup of water; or a teaspoon of peppermint tea every ten minutes until the symptoms subside. Peppermint bath is excellent for acute digestive disorders, tension, and anxiety. Make 2 quarts of triple strength tea (1 to 2 tablespoons per cup placed in a hot bath), or you may immerse 2 tea bags of peppermint tea in a bath tub, or simply add 1 teaspoon of peppermint oil into a hot bath. Some persons with digestive disorders carry the oil or teabags with them wherever they go. Be careful not to use peppermint tea that is blended with black tea, as black tea contains caffeine.

Chamomile

I consider chamomile a weaker version of peppermint, although others find it more soothing and less stimulating. It is traditionally used for nervousness and anxiety. It may also be used for intestinal spasms, mild acid indigestion and intestinal gas. Use one tea bag or a teaspoon of the herb steeped in boiling water. It may also be applied topically as per the instructions for peppermint.

Digestive Harmony

Digestive Harmony is a digestive tonic that I developed based on the traditional Chinese formula *Bao He Wan*. It is used for diarrhea, "traveler's stomach," and food stagnation associated with overeating. Digestive Harmony tablets can be chewed after meals to enhance digestion, or between meals for abdominal fullness, flatulence, or queasiness. General dosage is 2 tablets with meals, or 3 times per day. Digestive Harmony contains poria *(Fu Ling)*, coix *(Yi Yi Ren)*, Barley Shen Chu *(Shen Qu)*, magnolia bark *(Hou Po)*, angelica *(Bai Zhi)*, pueraria *(Ge Gen)*, red atractylodes *(Cang Zhu)*, vladimiria souliei *(Mu Xiang)*, pogostemon *(Huo Xiang)*, oryza *(Gu Ya)*, trichosanthes root *(Tian Hua Fen)*, chrysanthemum *(Ju Hua)*, halloysite *(Chi Shi Zhi)*, and red citrus *(Ju Hong)*.

Pau D'Arco

Pau D'Arco is an ancient Brazilian herb taken from the inner bark of the lapacho trees (*Tabebuia avellanedae*). I have had excellent reports on its effectiveness for candidiasis, including oral thrush. The dosage is 5 to 8 cups per day. There may be differences in quality among various suppliers. The alcohol extract is not as strong as the tea, and is not recommended for treatment of candidiasis.

Fennel

Over two thousand years ago, Hippocrates prescribed fennel for infants with colic. Fennel is used by both Chinese and American herbalists for the treatment of digestive disorders. Either chew a handful of seeds, use it as a spice in cooking, or use the powder, (1 to 2 teaspoons boiled for 5 minutes, steeped for another 10 minutes, then strained). If used for colic, use ⅓ the adult dosage.

Marjoram

Marjoram is a common spice that has been used in America since colonial times to treat infantile colic and as a digestant, tranquilizer, and cough remedy. Marjoram appears to soothe the digestive tract. Combine it with food, or take 1 to 2 teaspoons of dried leaves and flowers per cup of boiling water. Boil for 4 minutes and steep for another 10 minutes. Drink up to 3 cups a day.

Radish

Use a press or juicer to make juice from whole radishes; consume ½ to ⅔ cup of juice per day to gently stimulate peristalsis. You may also simply eat one whole radish several times a day. Radishes are traditionally use for dyspepsia, chronic constipation, and chronic gallbladder inflammation. If you cannot tolerate radishes try another remedy.

Kitchen Pharmacy

These items may be used as spices in cooking, or as infusions. You may also find essential oils of these spices for external use in your health food store.

Aniseed: flatulence, nervousness

Basil: anxiety, nervous insomnia

Bergamot: antispasmodic

Chamomile: loss of appetite

Caraway: indigestion

Clove: indigestion, diarrhea, nervousness

Coriander: indigestion

Cumin: nervousness

Cypress: hemorrhoids (applied topically)

Fennel: intestinal gas, stomach pain, indigestion, nervousness

Geranium: gastroenteritis, diarrhea

Ginger: indigestion, intestinal gas, loss of appetite

Lavender: stress, spasm, insomnia

Lemon: ulcers, intestinal parasites, diarrhea

Lemongrass: indigestion, nervousness

Lime peel: nervousness

Marjoram: intestinal gas, nervousness

Nutmeg: indigestion, diarrhea, intestinal gas

Onion: indigestion, diarrhea, parasites, nervousness

Orange blossom: chronic diarrhea, insomnia

Orange peel: nervousness

Origanum: loss of appetite, indigestion, intestinal gas

Parsley: nervousness

Peppermint: indigestion, intestinal gas, spasm, nervousness

Rosemary: colitis, intestinal infections, stomachache, liver disorders, jaundice, gallstones, cirrhosis, cholecystitis

Sage: tonic, indigestion, diarrhea, nervousness

Sandalwood: chronic diarrhea

Savory: indigestion, nervousness affecting digestive system, parasites

Spearmint: nervousness

Tarragon: indigestion, loss of appetite, intestinal gas

Terebinth: spasms, chronic constipation

Thyme: nervousness, indigestion, intestinal parasites

Ylang-ylang: intestinal infections

Herbs That Can Be Self-Administered With Some Caution

Ginger

Ginger was used as a digestant by the ancient Romans, and today is frequently employed by Western and Asian herbalists. Ginger contains digestive enzymes, anti-ulcer constituents, as well as pain-relieving, anti-inflammatory, and circulation-enhancing properties. As ginger is a warming herb, it is more suitable for people who feel cold, or whose health worsens in cold, damp weather (see "Cold Condition," Chapter One). It is contraindicated for people who feel hot or have a fever. Powdered ginger may be combined with food, or for stronger effects take ¼ teaspoon of powdered ginger and add it to 1 cup of boiling water to make a tea. Over time you may be able to increase your dosage of the powder to ½ teaspoon. Powdered ginger is much stronger than the fresh herb. In a pinch you can use fresh ginger by taking a teaspoon of freshly grated ginger and boiling it for 5 or 10 minutes before drinking.

Slippery Elm

Slippery elm is traditionally used to coat, protect, and rejuvenate the stomach and intestines. It is used to treat both constipation and diarrhea. Herbalists recommend slippery elm for the treatment of ulcers, colitis, and diverticulitis, i.e., any condition that involves inflammation. For acute gastrointestinal inflammation, add 1 teaspoon of slippery elm to a cup of hot or lukewarm water; and take it 4 to 5 times per day. Herbalists sometimes combine 3 parts slippery elm with 1 part comfrey root powder to treat gastric or intestinal inflammation and ulcers. (Comfrey root is not recommended for long-term administration because it contains active ingredients that may be harmful to the liver.) For those with cold signs, 3 parts slippery elm can be combined with 1 part ginger powder. I recommend slippery elm along with more powerful circulatory formulas, such as Isatis Cooling for hot conditions or Flavonex when hot signs are absent.

Hops

Hops have been traditionally used since ancient times for insomnia, restlessness, and diarrhea. Modern research indicates that hops relax smooth muscles and are a sedative. They have reportedly been used to treat digestive disorders, particularly IBS and colitis. Some herbalists suggest using the fresh herb as a digestive aid, and dried, aged hops as a sedative. Hops are consumed as a tea several times per day by using 2 teaspoons of herb per cup of boiling water, then steeping for 5 minutes. Hops are not recommended for people suffering from depression.

Valerian

Ancient Greek physicians including Dioscorides recommended valerian for nausea and for digestive and liver problems. The herb has been commonly used in Europe and America. Modern researchers have confirmed the efficacy of valerian for insomnia and in the treatment of anxiety. Western herbalists often combine it with herbs such as passion flower and lemon balm. The dosage is usually between 200 and 1,000 mg per dose. For tinctures, follow the directions on the bottle.

Some individuals may find valerian causes emotional aggravation in which case it should be discontinued. This is often seen in persons with hot conditions (see Chapter One). Valerian is an example of an adjunctive herb that can be used for people whose digestive disorder seems to be related to the nervous system, especially those with IBS.

Yarrow

Yarrow stimulates digestion, and can be taken 10 minutes before eating by those who have poor appetites. This herb also treats indigestion, and is said to have anti-inflammatory and anti-homeostatic (anti-bleeding) properties. Drink as a tea, by steeping 1 to 2 teaspoons in 1 cup of hot water for 20 minutes; take 2 to 8 cups a day.

Goldenseal

Goldenseal helps soothe the gastrointestinal system, and is used for its antibiotic properties in the gastrointestinal system. For this herb to be effective, symptoms of heat must be evident. Goldenseal should not be used by persons with cold conditions because in such cases taking this herb can weaken the health, therefore I recommend against self-prescribing unless it is for a cold or the flu (see Echinacea and Goldenseal later in this chapter).

Bitters

Bitters contain gentian and other ingredients useful for stimulating digestion. Gentian is still used today in liqueurs and vermouth. According to Chinese medicine, gentian should not be taken alone or in combination with other bitters, nor should it be taken in large dosages or on a daily basis, unless recommended by your health professional, because it is too cooling in nature and may cause diarrhea.

Flax

Flax lubricates and soothes the intestines. It is beneficial in the prevention and treatment of constipation. Use 1 to 2 tablespoons, 2 to 3 times per day, of flax oil added to vegetables or salad; or 1 to 2 tablespoons of freshly crushed seeds twice per day with hot water.

Dandelion

Dandelion is used in both Chinese and Western herbal medicines. Western herbalists often recommend dandelion as a spring tonic. This herb is thought to benefit the liver and gallbladder and to have a diuretic effect. To make an infusion, add 1 to 2 teaspoons of the crushed root to a cup of water, boil briefly, and allow it to sit covered for 15 minutes. One cup is taken every evening for 4 to 6 weeks. Dandelion juice can be taken 1 to 2 tablespoons per day in half a glass of water. Chinese herbalists consider dandelion too cold for routine use, unless hot signs are present.

Echinacea and Goldenseal

These are important cold- and flu-fighting herbs. The reason they are mentioned in this book is if that when taken during the first stages of a cold or the flu, you may be able to avoid becoming sick, or the symptoms may be lessened. Using these herbs in the initial stages of a cold or flu will also reduce your need for antibiotics; however, if your condition does not improve within a few days, see a health professional.

The best way to take these herbs is together in pill form; the usual dosage is 3 pills (500 to 750 mg) 3 to 6 times a day. I have formulated a product called Isatis Gold, which combines echinacea, goldenseal, and isatis. The latter is an herb that has antiviral and antibacterial properties. If, for instance, you have a cold or the flu, but are not running a fever, you may combine Echinacea and Goldenseal formula with freshly grated ginger tea. The tea is made by cutting 3 or 4 slices of fresh ginger, boiling for about 5 minutes before drinking. Contrary to the advice you receive in some health food stores, echinacea is a short-term herb, only to be taken before or during a cold or the flu. This herb or its products should not be taken for more than 10 days at a time. An alternate cold and flu remedy is a formula famous in China called *Yin Chao,* which is beneficial for the early stages of a cold or the flu. Make sure to use brands manufactured in America, as many of the Chinese brands contain pharmaceuticals.

Garlic

Garlic can be taken raw, or in its odorless form. It is used to combat yeast overgrowth, and is said to benefit the immune and circulatory systems, and to aid in the reduction of high cholesterol. Whether raw or cooked, Chinese medicine considers garlic to be warming, therefore it is not suitable for long-term administration if signs of heat are present. Odorless garlic, however, appears to be not as warming. Garlic may benefit some people, but is an irritant to others. Therefore, do not take garlic every day without the supervision of a knowledgeable herbalist.

Fresh garlic seems to be an effective anti-parasitic compound and has been used in Chinese medicine for thousands of years. Fresh garlic preparation is made by peeling 30 fresh cloves. Combine with a small amount of water in a blender, processing for short periods until the garlic and water are homogenized. Keep

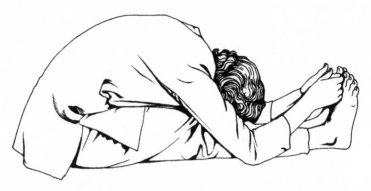

Posterior Stretch
This exercise is especially beneficial for the digestive system. Sit with your head, neck, and trunk straight, and your legs stretched in front of your body. When inhaling, raise your arms overhead, stretching toward the sky and expanding the chest as your breath fills your lungs. When exhaling, bend forward as far as possible while keeping your back straight and your knees on the floor; hold this position for 5 to 10 seconds. To be effective, this exercise should be repeated 20 or more times.

the garlic mixture chilled. Take 1 part garlic to 20 parts distilled water. Consume ⅓ to ½ cup of the mixture 2 to 3 times per day. Whole garlic cloves can also be chewed and swallowed with water. In a clinical study conducted in Egypt, stool samples of children who received the above garlic mixture for 3 days showed that giardia, a common parasite, was completely eliminated in all subjects.[1]

Milk Thistle *(Sylibum marianum)*

Milk thistle is a plant in the daisy family. Traditionally it was used as a digestive bitter; today it is regarded as one of the best liver herbs. The seeds contain an active ingredient called silymarin, which has been proven to have liver protection effects in animal experiments. Specifically, it protects the liver from adverse cellular changes and reduces fats in the liver. In Europe, an injection of milk thistle is used to treat people suffering from the potentially fatal Amanita mushroom poisoning. When silymarin is given to patients with chronic hepatitis, improvement is usually seen within the first two weeks of treatment. Patients experience less epigastric tension, improved appetite and physical performance. Silymarin acts on the membranes of the liver cells, preventing the entry of virus and other toxic compounds. Milk thistle and its products have been helpful in treating acute hepatitis, cirrhosis, and alcohol-damaged liver, and can be taken to offset the effects of liver-destructive pharmaceuticals.

I have been using a formula called Ecliptex, which contains milk thistle and other liver protective and regenerating herbs such as curcuma and schizandra, and is effective for the abovementioned conditions, especially when taken with the anti-toxin compound Clear Heat. General dosage is 2 to 3 tablets of Ecliptex, plus 1 to 3 tablets of Clear Heat, 3 times per day. A higher dosage of Clear Heat is indicated for heat signs.

You can also take powered extracts of milk thistle (400 to 500 mg per day for 4 to 6 weeks, then reduce to 100 mg per day), or take 1 teaspoon of crushed seeds with hot water, 4 times per day. Powdered extracts of milk thistle are available over the counter, either alone or combined with ingredients such as dandelion, rhubarb, artichoke, ox bile, and choline.

Laxative Tea Home Remedy

Add 1 teaspoon each of caraway seed, fennel seed, peppermint leaves, senna leaves, and chamomile to 1 quart of water (approximately 1 liter), infuse for 15 minutes, and consume 1 cup, morning and night. If this mixture is too strong for you, reduce the dosage or omit the senna leaves.

Herbs That Should Only Be Administered by a Practitioner

Licorice

Numerous studies have shown that licorice is an effective anti-ulcer compound. It has also been shown to reduce gastric bleeding caused by aspirin, therefore it is a good preventive of gastric ulcer in patients who are taking aspirin and other non-steroidal anti-inflammatory medications. Licorice is as effective as pharmaceuticals such as cimetidine (Tagamet) and ranitidine (Zantac), and some studies have found that it is more effective than antacids. Licorice is a common ingredient in Chinese herbal formulas such as Six Gentlemen and Stomach Tabs. There are reports of licorice causing side effects such as headaches and high blood pressure; however, such symptoms occur only when licorice root is taken by itself in large doses (over 5 g per day). As one of several ingredients in a Chinese herbal formula, this herb is not harmful, nor is deglycyrrhizinic acid (DGL), a special licorice compound that must be chewed.

Isatis Cooling

I developed this formula to treat ulcers, as well as Crohn's disease and ulcerative colitis. Isatis Cooling has been used by thousands of patients struggling with digestive disorders, especially when pain is an accompanying symptom. This formula has anti-inflammatory, anti-toxin, and blood circulating ingredients. Most individuals using this formula notice that it reduces the burning and stabbing pain associated with gastrointestinal flare ups. I have had reports that some persons have been able to avoid colon surgery after using this remedy. The ingredients are: isatis extract *(Ban Lan Gen* and *Da Qing Ye)*, codonopsis *(Dang Shen)*, oyster shell *(Mu Li)*, bupleurum *(Chai Hu)*, smilax *(Tu Fu Ling)*, gardenia *(Zhi Zi)*, moutan *(Mu Dan Pi)*, tang-kuei *(Dang Gui)*, akebia *(Mu Tong)*, red peony *(Chi Shao)*, alisma *(Ze Xie)*, cyperus *(Xiang Fu)*. In terms of TCM, Isatis Cooling clears heat and toxins and circulates blood. General dosage is 3 to 5 tablets, 3 times per day.

Six Gentlemen (Modified)

Modified Six Gentlemen with vladimiria souliei and cardamon is a very beneficial tonic for people with digestive disorders, since invariably a weak digestive system is either the root of the problem or is a result of the gastrointestinal disease. This historical formula addresses fatigue, nausea, loss of appetite, and bloating and is a follow up treatment to formulas such as Isatis Cooling. The ingredients are: codonopsis *(Dang Shen)*, white atractylodes *(Bai Zhu)*, poria *(Fu Ling)*, baked licorice *(Zhi Gan Cao)*, citrus *(Chen Pi)*, pinellia *(Ban Xia)*, vladimiria souliei *(Mu Xiang)*, cardamon *(Sha Ren)*. In terms of TCM, Six Gentlemen tonifies Qi, transforms phlegm, and harmonizes the spleen/stomach. General dosage is 3 tablets, 3 times per day.

Source Qi

This formula is based on the traditional Chinese remedy *Sheng Qi Shi Zang Wan* (Raise the Qi and Consolidate the Organs Pill). The indications for usage are diarrhea accompanied by sinking of Source Qi, extreme deficiency of the spleen/stomach, prolapse of the anus, and loss of appetite. Other symptoms that can be addressed by this formula are food not being digested, fluids not being absorbed and "passing straight through," extreme thirst, insufficient fluids, weight loss and wasting of the limbs, and fever and chills. Source Qi can be taken for chronic deficiency accompanied by cold signs, and is used mainly for conditions in which long-term diarrhea is present, such as in Crohn's disease, cancer, and chronic parasitic, viral, or bacterial infections. It is generally not used for conditions that have heat signs. The ingredients are: ailanthus *(Chun Bai Pi)*, baked astragalus *(Huang Qi)*, white ginseng *(Ren Shen)*, white atractylodes *(Bai Zhu)*, red atractylodes *(Cang Zhu)*, poria *(Fu Ling)*, dioscorea *(Shan Yao)*, lotus seed *(Lian Zi)*, euryale *(Qian Shi)*, cimicifuga *(Sheng Ma)*, fried bupleurum *(Chai Hu)*, charcoaled ginger *(Gan Jiang)*, nutmeg *(Rou Dou Kou)*, baked licorice *(Zhi Gan Cao)*, barley shen qu *(Shen Qu)*. In terms of TCM, Source Qi strengthens the spleen/stomach, astringes fluids, tonifies Qi, and improves digestive function. General dosage is 3 to 5 tablets 3 times per day.

Quiet Digestion

This formula treats gastric distress, including abdominal pain, sudden and violent cramping, nausea, vomiting, diarrhea, regurgitation, gastric hyperactivity, intestinal gas, abdominal distention, and poor appetite. It is a safe and versatile remedy that is taken with meals to help food assimilate, and between meals for the abovementioned symptoms. In cases of food poisoning or extreme (violent) symptoms it is helpful to crush 1 to 2 tablets and add to fresh ginger tea (see this chapter). The ingredients are: poria *(Fu Ling)*, coix *(Yi Yi Ren)*, barley shen chu *(Shen Qu)*, magnolia bark *(Hou Po)*, angelica *(Bai Zhi)*, pueraria *(Ge Gen)*, red atractylodes *(Cang Zhu)*, vladimiria souliei *(Mu Xiang)*, pogostemon *(Huo Xiang)*, oryza *(Gu Ya)*, trichosanthes root *(Tian Hua Fen)*, chrysanthemum *(Ju Hua)*, halloysite *(Chi Shi Zhi)*, red citrus *(Ju Hong)*. In terms of TCM, Quiet Digestion disperses wind and dampness, resolves spleen dampness and regulates the stomach, and resolves phlegm. General dosage is 2 tablets every few hours for acute cases; 2 to 3 tablets 3 times per day for chronic conditions; or 1 tablet before and 1 tablet after meals to help food assimilate.

Stomach Tabs

This remedy improves digestion, resolves flatulence, relieves abdominal bloating, soothes acute and chronic gastritis, and treats gastric ulcer. Since this is a warming formula, it is used to treat conditions that are accompanied by cold signs. For heat signs with similar symptoms, use Isatis Cooling (see this chapter). The ingredients are: magnolia bark *(Hou Po)*, citrus *(Chen Pi)*, pinellia *(Ban Xia)*, red atractylodes *(Cang Zhu)*, ginger *(Gan Jiang)*, licorice *(Gan Cao)*, bupleurum *(Chai Hu)*, oryza *(Gu Ya)*. In terms of TCM, Stomach Tabs disperses stagnant Qi, resolves spleen dampness, dispels food stagnation, and resolves stomach phlegm. General dosage is: 2 to 3 tablets, 3 times per day.

Formula H

This formula reduces inflammation of hemorrhoidal tissues, stops bleeding, and resolves bloody stools due to other conditions. I have used this formula successfully (in conjunction with Western medical diagnosis and treatment) along with Colostroplex (see this chapter) to treat bloody stools due to ulcerative colitis and Crohn's disease. The ingredients are: sanguisorba *(Di Yu)*, pulsatilla *(Bai Tou Weng)*, sophora flower *(Huai Hua Mi)*, white peony

(Bai Shao), tang-kuei *(Dang Gui)*, rehmannia *(Sheng Di Huang)*, fraxinus *(Qin Pi)*, phellodendron *(Huang Bai)*, lonicera *(Jin Yin Hua)*. In terms of TCM, Formula H clears heat and eliminates dampness, nourishes the blood and promotes circulation, consolidates Yin, stops bleeding. General dosage is 3 to 5 tablets, 3 times per day.

Before using this formula, patients should undergo a thorough biomedical diagnosis, because bleeding can be caused by cancer or other serious disease.

Phellostatin

I developed Phellostatin in alliance with a biochemist over ten years ago to treat candidiasis, which is often a contributing factor in digestive disorders, and to treat sinus congestion, skin rashes, vaginal itching, and lethargy. Phellostatin may be considered a Chinese herbal "colon cleanser," and many of its herbs have antifungal effects. Patients who have longstanding digestive disorders with heat, may take a combination of Phellostatin and Isatis Cooling. With weakness and cold signs combine Phellostatin with Six Gentlemen; with intestinal gas and bloating, combine Phellostatin with Quiet Digestion. The ingredients are: phellodendron *(Huang Bai)*, codonopsis *(Dang Shen)*, white atractylodes *(Bai Zhu)*, anemarrhena *(Zhi Mu)*, plantago *(Che Qian Zi)*, pulsatilla *(Bai Tou Weng)*, capillaris *(Yin Chen Hao)*, cnidium fruit *(She Chuang Zi)*, houttuynia *(Yu Xing Cao)*, dioscorea *(Shan Yao)*, licorice *(Gan Cao)*, cardamon *(Sha Ren)*. In terms of TCM, Phellostatin tonifies spleen/stomach Qi and resolves damp-heat. Dosage during the first week of starting this formula is 1 tablet, 3 times per day; thereafter, the dosage is 2 to 3 tablets, 3 times per day.

Flavonex

Flavonex is a formula that increases circulation and has anti-inflammatory properties. One of its many ingredients is ginkgo, which comes from the oldest living tree species. Ginkgo and other herbs such as salvia are often used in the treatment of seniors and those who have circulatory disorders such as impaired memory and intermittent claudication (pain or weakness of the calf or foot when walking). This formula treats digestive disorders due to poor circulation, particularly conditions involving ulcers, such as gastric ulcers, ulcerative colitis, Crohn's disease. The ingredients are: pueraria *(Ge Gen)*, ilex *(Mao Dong Qing)*, salvia *(Dan Shen)*, lonicera *(Jin Yin Hua)*, eucommia *(Du Zhong)*, acorus *(Shi Chang Pu)*, cistanche *(Rou Cong Rong)*, ho-shou-wu *(He Shou Wu)*, morus fruit *(Sang Shen)*, rose fruit *(Jin Ying Zi)*, lycium fruit *(Gou Qi Zi)*, zizyphus *(Suan Zao Ren)*, tang-kuei *(Dang Gui)*, schizandra *(Wu Wei Zi)*, gingko biloba extract *(Yin Guo Ye)*. In terms of TCM, Flavonex promotes circulation of Qi and blood, and tonifies the kidney. General dosage is 3 to 4 tablets, 3 times per day.

Ginkgo

In addition to treating circulatory conditions, ginkgo biloba has also been found to be effective in treating digestive disorders. In a clinical study, ten patients with IBD between the ages of 35 and 75 were given retention enemas containing 200 mg of standardized ginkgo biloba mixed in 4 ounces of water. The enemas were administered before bedtime and the patients were told to retain this mixture throughout the night. After three weeks, three patients experienced complete remission, two reported improvement, and five showed no change. Perhaps better results may be obtained by combining ginkgo enemas with herbal formulas containing ginkgo, such as Flavonex.

Robert's Formula

This is a classic American herbal formula consisting of marshmallow root, *Geranium maculatim,* goldenseal, echinacea, and pokeweed *(Phytolacca decandra).* Slippery elm and okra are sometimes added. American herbalists use this formula to treat ulcers. It can be combined with calming agents such as hops, passionflower, and mint. General dosage is: 4 to 9 capsules or tablets per day.

Bilberry

Bilberry tea or extract treats diarrhea especially due to an infection, as the blue pigment most likely inhibits bacterial growth. Bilberry can also be used to treat dyspepsia and diarrhea in infants. Bilberry is said to be astringent, antiseptic, and absorptive. Its tea is made by boiling 3 tablespoons for 10 minutes in ½ quart (½ liter) of water, and then taking a glass of the strained liquid several times throughout the day.

Shepherd's Purse

Shepherd's purse *(Capsuella bursa-pastoris)* stops bleeding of the stomach, bowels, lungs, and vagina. I recommend using the powdered herb, while others report good results with the tincture. General dosage is: 6 to 9 tablets (3 to 4.5 grams) daily.

Before using this remedy, patients should undergo a thorough biomedical diagnosis, because bleeding can be caused by cancer and other serious disease.

Anti-Parasitic Formulas

For clients who are infected with multiple parasites, I recommend a protocol of Artestatin and Aquilaria 22 to be taken for two months, followed by Biocidin and Six Gentlemen for one month. Black walnut hulls may also be used for an additional month. **Always begin anti-parasitic herbs at a reduced dosage to avoid unpleasant reactions.** These remedies are discussed below.

Artestatin

This formula is made up of several anti-parasitic herbs, including *Artemesia anua (Qing Hao)* and the special ingredient brucea, which kills amoebae in the cyst stage. Artestatin is used alone to treat protozoal infections such as giardiasis. For a more broad spectrum effect, combine Artestatin with Aquilaria 22, the general dosage being 1 to 3 tablets of Artestatin, 3 times per day, and 1 to 2 tablets of Aquilaria 22, 3 times per day. For diarrhea, decrease the dosage of Aquilaria 22, and for constipation, increase Aquilaria 22. The ingredients of Artestatin are: artemisia anua concentrate *(Qing Hao)*, dichroa *(Chang Shan)*, Brucea *(Yu Dan Zi)*, pulsatilla *(Bai Tou Weng)*, magnolia bark *(Hou Po)*, pinellia *(Ban Xia)*, pogostemon *(Huo Xiang)*, dolichos *(Bai Bian Dou)*, codonopsis *(Dan Shen)*, citrus *(Chen Pi)*, licorice *(Gan Cao)*, coptis *(Huang Lian)*, red atractylodes *(Cang Zhu)*, ginger *(Gan Jiang)*, cardamon *(Sha Ren)*. In terms of TCM, Artestatin clears summer heat, expels parasites, and promotes the circulation of Qi.

Aquilaria 22

This is a compound of herbs traditionally used in the treatment of parasites, worms, and chronic constipation. The ingredients are: aquilaria *(Chen Xiang)*, ginger *(Gan Jiang)*, mume *(Wu Mei)*, codonopsis *(Dang Shen)*, terminalia *(He Zi)*, poria *(Fu Ling)*, white atractylodes *(Bai Zhu)*, quisqualis *(Shi Jun Zi)*, omphalia *(Lei Wan)*, vladimiria souliei *(Mu Xiang)*, torreya *(Fei Zi)*, areca *(Da Fu Pi)*, pomegranate *(Shi Liu Pi)*, melia *(Chuan Lian Zi)*, rubus *(Fu Pen Zi)*, aurantium *(Zhi Shi)*, nutmeg *(Rou Dou Kou)*, white cardamon *(Bai Dou Kou)*, ulmus *(Wu Yi)*, zanthoxylum *(Chuan Jiao)*, licorice *(Gan Cao)*, aloe *(Lu Hui)*. In terms of TCM, Aquilaria 22 purges Gallbladder heat and moves Qi.

Biocidin (Gentiana Formula)

Biocidin (Gentiana Formula) is a potent combination of Chinese and Western herbs, including chlorophyll and garlic. It has anti-parasitic, antibacterial, and anti-fungal properties. Instructions: During the first week, add 1 to 2 drops of Biocidin to a few ounces of water, juice, or on a cracker with meals. As per tolerance, gradually increase over the course of 2 to 3 weeks to 4 to 5 drops. Do not use more than 4 to 5 drops at a time, and do not exceed 15 drops per day total. The average course is 6 to 12 weeks; however, this may vary accordingly to individual needs. It is not usually necessary to stay at the maximum dosage (15 drops per day) for more than 4 to 8 weeks; a maintenance dosage of 3 to 9 drops total per day should suffice. Biocidin tablets may be taken as directed on the label. This remedy should be taken with the formula Six Gentlemen and acidophilus/bifidus supplements. Six Gentlemen counters the cooling property of Biocidin and acidophilus/bifidus restores the health gut bacteria, which is often disrupted during parasitic infections. The ingredients of Biocidin are: chlorophyll, Impatiens pallida, Hydrastis canadensis, Ferula galbanum, Hypericum perforatum, Villa rubris, Frasera carolinensis, Gentiana campestris, fumaria, sanguinaria, allicin, garlic.

Black Walnut Hulls

Black walnut hulls can be a part of anti-parasitic or anti-worm therapy. I recommend this product be taken in capsule form, starting at 1 capsule per day, up to 5 capsules, 3 times per day. Some people report cramping and diarrhea with this herb, so it must be used carefully; however, it may be worth the risk for parasite infections that are not responding to other therapies. An herbalist friend of mine contracted parasites in Indonesia that were drug-resistant. After a several-month course of Chinese herbs (Artestatin and Aquilaria 22), she took black walnut hulls in capsule form and was free of the parasites within several months.

Vitamins and Dietary Supplements

Patients with chronic digestive disorders may have long-standing deficiencies of basic nutrients due to chronic malabsorption. In addition, digestive diseases and medications used to treat these diseases may increase the need for nutrients. Nutrients work as a team; not getting enough of one nutrient may reduce the efficacy of its co-factors. Supplements are very beneficial to patients with digestive disorders. Antioxidants are of particular importance, because they help repair and protect the body against cellular damage.

It is important to note that people with digestive disorders can have sensitivities. For example, one of my clients had a reaction to B vitamins and even became ill after taking multiple B vitamins. Another client had a reaction to iron supplementation despite being anemic (he had to rely on meat for iron). Likewise, it may be necessary to try different brands before finding the ones that work well for you. This section lists helpful vitamins, minerals, and special dietary supplements.

Daily Supplement Plan for Digestive Disorders

Look for a single supplement that is a broad spectrum antioxidant containing beta-carotene or mixed carotenoids, vitamin C, vitamin E, zinc, and selenium. I use a supplement called Quercenol, which contains added cofactors. If you cannot find a product with the dosages listed below, buy the single supplements.

- **Beta-carotene**—starting dosage is 10,000 IU; increase to 50,000 IU per day, or use products with mixed carotenoids (30 mg per day)
- **Vitamin C**—(calcium ascorbate-ester C may be easier to digest) 500 mg to 2,000 mg per day
- **Vitamin E**—200 to 800 IU per day
- **Selenium**—50 mcg to 200 mcg per day
- **Zinc**—10 mg to 50 mg per day (you may need to experiment with brands)

Tip

Always take the following nutrients with meals. Start at the lowest dosage and gradually increase. The dosage of a vitamin is much more individual than even experts admit. Therefore, some people will notice a definite health improvement after 4 to 8 weeks at the low dosage, while in others it may take up to 6 months at the highest dosage.

- **Vitamin B**$_{12}$—250 to 1,000 mcg per day
- **Folic acid**—400 mcg to 800 mcg per day

Other nutrients that may be included:

- **L-Cysteine**—100 mg to 1,000 mg per day
- **Multiple B vitamin formula**—(eliminate if symptoms worsen)
- **Max EPA**—fish oil capsules (for Crohn's disease or ulcerative colitis, see "Fish Oil" section, later in this chapter)
- **Quercetin**—300 mg to 2,000 mg per day
- **Minerals**—Calcium/magnesium used to reduce spasms. Calcium may be constipating; magnesium helps treat constipation; adjust dosage if symptoms, i.e., constipation or diarrhea, occur. Typical daily dosages: calcium—1,000 mg; magnesium—500 mg; if constipation is experienced, take equal amounts of both minerals.

Vitamin A
and Beta-Carotene

The role of vitamin A in maintaining normal vision was established nearly one hundred years ago. Since then, research has found that this vitamin has other important biological functions such as controlling normal cell development, enhancing the immune system, preventing certain cancers, and regulating the aging process. Dietary vitamin A is obtained directly from animal products such as milk, egg yolks, fish, and liver. It can also be derived from beta-carotene, one of the constituents in the family of pigments called carotenoids, which are found in plants and microorganisms. Beta-carotene is the predominant carotenoid in certain fruits and vegetables such as carrots, spinach, broccoli, sweet potatoes, cantaloupe, and pumpkin, among others, and is converted mainly in the liver and intestine to various forms of vitamin A called retinols. Some retinols contribute to skin and ligament repair, others to transporting enzymes and proteins, yet others to the bioelectrical process of vision. Carotenoids have antioxidant properties, acting as free-radical scavengers in eliminating damaged cells in our bodies. Therefore, these micronutrients are particularly important for patients with IBD (Crohn's disease and ulcerative colitis), since such individuals are at increased likelihood of developing colon cancer. Vegetables and fruits that are rich in carotenoids should be eaten every day. Even with sufficient fruits and vegetables at every meal, supplementation with beta-carotene is highly recommended.

Vitamin A can be toxic at high doses, whereas large doses of beta-carotene are not. Therefore, it is advisable to obtain supplemental vitamin A by taking beta-carotene or mixed carotenoids so as to avoid risk of vitamin toxicity. Pregnant women should not take more than 5,000 IU of vitamin A, because large doses can cause birth defects. Antibiotics, laxatives, and cholesterol-lowering drugs interfere with vitamin A absorption. Also, diabetics and individuals suffering from hyperthyroidism cannot convert beta-carotene to vitamin A, therefore if you use the preceding medications or have these disorders, consult your health professional about supplementing with vitamin A.

Vitamin E

This is another antioxidant that is thought to prevent cancer and cardiovascular disease, support the immune system, and promote cell repair. Holistic practitioners recommend the use of vitamin E to improve circulation, treat digestive disorders, reduce blood pressure, promote clotting and healing, reduce scarring, and relieve leg cramps. Vitamin E works synergistically with vitamin C, thus these two supplements should be taken together.

Vitamin C

Vitamin C protects against blood clotting and bruising, and promotes the healing of wounds. It is also important for proper adrenal gland functioning, and since the latter is most affected by high levels of stress, vitamin C helps the body in recovering from and protection against stress. Aspirin and other analgesics, alcohol, antidepressants, anticoagulants, contraceptives, and steroids may reduce the levels of vitamin C in the body. Those who have trouble digesting regular vitamin C might want to use the more expensive ester C or try buffered vitamin C.

Zinc

Zinc is important for a healthy immune system and for promoting wound healing. This mineral is required for protein synthesis and collagen formation. Zinc levels may be lowered by conditions such as diarrhea, kidney disease, cirrhosis of the liver, and diabetes. Dosages above 100 mg per day are not recommended. The two primary forms of zinc that holistic doctors prefer are zinc citrate and zinc picolinate.

Selenium

Selenium protects the immune system by preventing the formation of free radical scavengers. It is needed for pancreatic function and tissue elasticity.

Vitamin D

Vitamin D is important for calcium utilization, which helps build strong bones and protects against cancer. Dairy products and fatty fish contain vitamin D. If you do not eat these foods, you might consider supplementing with vitamin D.

The B Vitamins

B vitamins help maintain the muscle tone of the digestive tract and proper functioning of the nerves, therefore they may be useful in the treatment of depression and anxiety. Generally the B vitamins should be taken in combination. Perhaps the most important is B_{12}, followed by folic acid. These two are synergistic and should be taken together. Vitamin B_{12} prevents pernicious anemia, insures proper digestion and absorption, aids in the synthesis of protein and in the metabolism of carbohydrates and fat. Vitamin B_{12} deficiency may be caused by malabsorption and can lead to digestive disorders. Vegetarians have a special need for this vitamin. Anti-gout medications, anticoagulants, and potassium supplements can block the absorption of B_{12}.

Folic acid plays a vital role in the activities of various enzymes involved in the production of nucleic acids and thus in growth and reproduction. Therefore, a deficiency in folic acid can cause chromosomes to break at fragile places, allowing viruses to slip into the genetic material of healthy cells. Individuals with low levels of folic acid in their red blood cells are five times more likely to develop pre-cancerous cell changes than those with normal folic acid levels.

Vitamin B_1 (Thiamine) is important for proper blood circulation in that low levels of thiamine can result in sluggish circulation. This vitamin assists the body in the production of hydrochloric acid, in blood formation and carbohydrate metabolism. It is also needed to maintain the muscle tone of the stomach, intestines, and heart. Antibiotics, sulfa drugs (Azulfidine), and oral contraceptives decrease thiamin levels in the body.

Vitamin B$_2$ (riboflavin) is necessary for red blood cell formation, antibody production, cell respiration and growth. It also aids in the metabolism of carbohydrates, fats, and proteins. Vitamin B$_2$ works with vitamin A to maintain the mucous membrane of the digestive tract.

Vitamin B$_3$ (niacin, niacinamide, nicotinic acid) is needed for proper circulation and normal functioning of the nervous system. It also aids in the metabolism of carbohydrates, fats, and proteins and in the production of hydrochloric acid.

Vitamin B$_5$ (Pantothenic acid) is the premiere anti-stress vitamin. It is also important for the conversion of fats, carbohydrates, and proteins, into energy. A normal level of this vitamin assures the healthy functioning of the gastrointestinal tract. Holistic doctors recommend using vitamin B$_5$ to help patients wean themselves from steroid medications, as it is thought to stimulate the body's own cortisone production. Pantothenic acid also promotes wound healing, and treats constipation, fatigue, and stomach ulcers. People who have had part of their gastrointestinal tract removed need additional vitamin B$_5$, as do those with inadequate nutritional intake.

Vitamin B$_6$ (pyridoxine) helps the body produce hydrochloric acid and absorb fats and protein. It is also needed for the proper functioning of the nervous and immune systems, and for the reproduction of body cells. B$_6$ also activates many enzymes and aids in B$_{12}$ absorption. Antidepressants, estrogen, and oral contraceptives may increase the need for B$_6$.

Amino Acids

Amino acids are chemical compounds that serve as the building blocks of all proteins. Many biological processes are dependent upon proteins. There are twenty different amino acids that comprise all proteins in humans. Twelve of these can be made by the human body, and are known as nonessential amino acids because they do not need to be obtained from the diet. The other eight, the essential amino acids, must be obtained from the diet. The following amino acids are of particular importance to people with digestive conditions.

L-Cystine aids in the healing of burns and wounds. It also plays a role in fighting disease by promoting the function of white blood cells. L-cystine is necessary for the production of insulin, which is needed for the assimilation of sugars and starches.

L-Cysteine helps in the detoxification process, thus aiding in the protection of cells. Therefore, this amino acid is a powerful antioxidant. L-cysteine has the same benefits as L-cystine and is said to be helpful to those who suffer from rheumatoid arthritis.

L-Glutamine is said to help heal peptic ulcers and in the maintenance of a healthy digestive system. There is currently a debate with regard to the optimal dosage; some advocate 500 mg and others 1 teaspoon of the powder 3 times daily. Until the jury is in, I do not recommend this supplement.

L-Histidine is important for the production of red and white blood cells, and promotes healthy digestion and secretion of gastric juices. It is also said to be useful in the treatment of ulcers, allergies, rheumatoid arthritis, and anemia.

Calcium and Magnesium

Calcium and magnesium are important for many biological functions in the body. Calcium is necessary to keep teeth and bones healthy and strong. It also promotes blood coagulation and is essential in enabling muscles to relax and contract. Some research has suggested a relationship between calcium intake and colon cancer. Magnesium plays many roles in the body. It, too, is necessary for maintaining strong teeth and bones, and for helping the muscles work properly. Small amounts of magnesium have an antacid effect, while large amounts have a laxative effect. Calcium and magnesium can help relieve stress, and both have blood pressure–lowering effects. Long-term calcium deficiency can lead to osteoporosis, among other conditions; magnesium deficiency can cause impaired intestinal absorption, and possibly asthma and diabetes.

The RDA for calcium is 800 mg for men and women over the age of 25, with pregnant women needing an additional 400 mg per day. Many experts believe that we require more calcium than the official recommendation, up to 1,000 mg daily for premenopausal women, and 1,500 mg for postmenopausal women and seniors over 65.

For persons suffering abdominal spasms, regular supplementation with equal amounts of calcium and magnesium, or with one half as much magnesium as calcium, is advisable. Because these two minerals may be difficult to digest, when first starting supplementation, a reduced dosage should be used. Ask your healthcare professional about readily absorbable forms of calcium such as calcium citrate and calcium aspartate. I have formulated a product, called SPZM, that consists of calcium and magnesium in readily absorbable form, and is available through health professionals. It is designed to reduce spasms.

L. Acidophilus (Lactobacillus *acidophilus*)

Lactobacillus are a genus of bacteria that occur widely in nature and in the human mouth, vagina, and intestinal tract. *L. acidophilus,* and other "friendly" bacteria such as *B. bifidus* and *L. bulgaricus,* help protect us from unhealthy bacteria (see "Viral and Bacterial Infections," Chapter Four). As a supplement, *L. acidophilus* enhances digestion, helps correct lactose intolerance and resolve intestinal gas, promotes absorption of nutrients, and has antibacterial properties. In a study of hospitalized seniors who suffered constipation, subjects were given a daily dessert of *L. acidophilus* yogurt prune whip. Over 95 percent of the subjects no longer needed laxatives as long as they ate the special prune whip. Other effects of the *L. acidophilus* treatment were improvement in overall mental outlook and in diabetic ulcers for a number of patients who also suffered from diabetes.

In other studies, *L. acidophilus* was found to alleviate diarrhea in adults and infants, therefore it is recommended widely by herbalists and holistic doctors as a prophylactic while traveling in the third world. In a study conducted at Augsburg College in Minneapolis, subjects who took *L. acidophilus* capsules before traveling to Mexico, Nepal, and Guatemala reported no incidents of diarrhea or intestinal disorders, although their travel partners did.

L. acidophilus should be taken on an empty stomach so that it can become implanted in the intestines, thus it should be taken at bedtime and in the morning twenty minutes before consuming any food or drink. I recommend taking *L. acidophilus* with other healthy bacteria supplements such as *B. bifidus.* The products I have found to be of consistently good quality are PB 8, LGG, and Bacillus coagulans.

Colostroplex

Colostroplex is bovine colostrom freshly collected from six different herds of cattle. This product is aimed at restoring gastrointestinal function and is thought to improve gastrointestinal immunity, therefore it has many uses. I recommend Colostroplex for its anti-inflammatory, anti-viral, antibacterial/antifungal properties, in addition to its antidiarrheal action. Those who are sensitive to dairy products may find it helpful as well. For diarrhea, the dosage is 4 to 6 tablets daily; this dosage can be reduced as the stools become more formed. To ameliorate food sensitivities and allergies, use 1 to 2 tablets for 3 to 6 months. Reduce dosage if constipation occurs.

Bioflavonoids – Quercetin

Bioflavonoids are a group of compounds that are found widely in plants. For example, the white material just beneath the peel in citrus fruits is abundant in bioflavonoids. They are also found in peppers, buckwheat, and black currants. Bioflavonoids have antibacterial properties and help to maintain the strength of capillaries, promote circulation, and stimulate bile production. Bioflavonoids modify the body's response to inflammatory conditions such as arthritis, asthma, eczema, hayfever, and other allergies. They seem to work by inhibiting the release of histamine and other inflammatory compounds from mast cells, the tissues that are the usual site of allergic and inflammatory response.

Quercetin, a bioflavonoid that appears to have extensive therapeutic properties, is found in yellow and red onions, red grapes, broccoli, and Italian squash. It has anti-inflammatory, antibacterial, antifungal, and anti-viral properties. Recently, quercetin has come under extensive study for its anti-inflammatory properties. Specifically, this compound blocks the release of his-tamines, which cause the symptoms of typical allergic reactions such as hayfever and food allergies. To be effective, quercetin should be used for several months prior to allergy season.

Quercetin also inhibits the release of even stronger inflam-matory compounds such as leukotrienes, which contribute to the cause of psoriasis, gout, asthma, and ulcerative colitis, among other conditions. Quercetin can be taken with enzymes such as brome-lain to increase absorption. Recommended dosage for quercetin is 500 mg to 2,000 mg, taken several times throughout the day.

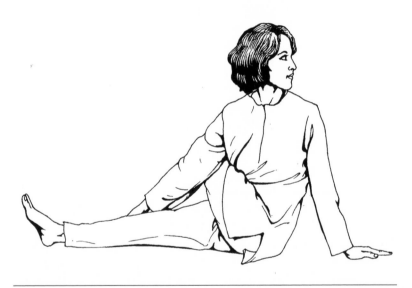

Half Spinal Twist
This exercise promotes circulation and digestion. Sit with your head, neck, and trunk straight, and your legs together. Bend your left leg, placing the left foot outside the right knee. Twist your body leftward and place your left hand 4 to 6 inches behind your left hip, fingers pointing away from the body. Bring your right arm over the outside of your left leg and grasp your left foot with your right hand. Keep your back straight, turn leftward, twisting the lower spine, and look over your left shoulder. Hold your breath for 5 seconds. Repeat with the opposite side. Perform this exercise at least 20 times.

For persons who do not take quercetin regularly, a dosage of 200 mg to 600 mg, 3 times per day, may be used to possibly prevent food sensitivity reactions.

Bromelain

Bromelain is an enzyme extracted from pineapple. It has protein-digesting and anti-inflammatory actions, and is used in the treatment of digestive disorders, trauma, arthritis, respiratory infections, scleroderma, and phlebitis. It is taken with meals to improve digestion, and between meals to reduce inflammation. Good quality bromelain has between 1,000 to 2,000 mcu (milk clotting units) per gram. It is recommended that you take products containing several enzymes, such as papain, trypsin, and chymotrypsin in addition to bromelain, because of their synergistic effects.

Fish Oil

Although fish oil has been studied for the treatment of IBD, results have been modest. In one study, eighteen patients received either eighteen capsules per day of Max EPA (fish oil) or vegetable oil capsules, for four months. Patients on the Max EPA were able to reduce their prednisone dosage by an average of 53 percent. There was also an improvement in bowel movement frequency among subjects in the fish oil group, as well as in weight gain.[3] I believe that by adding antioxidant vitamins, zinc, folic acid, and specific herbs to your program you can improve these results.

Enzymes

Proponents say that everyone, particularly those who do not eat raw foods, needs enzymes. I am not convinced because enzymes only break down food; they do not contribute to gastrointestinal healing as do herbs and other nutrients. I prefer to use Chinese herbal enzymes contained in remedies such as Digestive Harmony (Quiet Digestion), which is based on a formula used in China for over one hundred years.

However, for patients who cannot tolerate herbs, enzymes may in fact be the best compromise. For example, Beano™ is a commercially available enzyme product derived from the *Aspergillus* mold, which helps in the digestion of beans and cruciferous vegetables, such as cauliflower and broccoli. For digestive purposes, plant enzymes are recommended over the more common animal enzymes containing pancreatin and pepsin. Plant enzymes are able to survive any pH, whereas pancreatin, tyrosine, and chemotrypsin need acidity in order to be absorbed. In treating pancreatic and other cancers, plant enzymes such as papain and bromelain (proteolytic enzymes) are used to break down tumors. A dentist, William Kelly, is said to have cured his cancer using these enzymes. (The use of enzymes for treating cancer should be closely monitored by a health professional.)

If you are unable to find an herbalist to work with, you can experiment with taking 1 to 5 plant or proteolytic enzyme capsules before and after meals. Vegetable enzymes are usually taken with meals to help food assimilate, and because enzymes also have anti-inflammatory properties, they may be taken between meals for this purpose. A more cost-effective alternative to enzymes is to take hot ginger tea with a teaspoon of lime squeezed before each meal for cold conditions. If you have a hot condition, add cider vinegar to hot water or simply squeeze lemon or lime juice into a cup of hot water before meals. You can also drink peppermint tea before meals.

FOS

FOS stands for fructooligosaccharides, the carbohydrates found in small concentrations in many fruits, vegetables, and grains. One to two capsules, or ½ teaspoon or more powdered, of FOS can be taken per day on an empty stomach. FOS creates a less hospitable environment in the intestines for foreign bacteria by increasing the levels of good bacteria. It may be a good idea to take FOS along with acidophilus and bifidus at bedtime instead of a snack.

Caprylic Acid

Known by many different brand names, this is a saturated fatty acid used for treating candidiasis. Although there are usually no serious side effects from this product, based on the principles of Chinese medicine it has a warming effect, thus I do not recommend this remedy for candidiasis patients. In addition, it may cause gastrointestinal upset and a worsening of symptoms, as it causes yeast to be killed off.

Citrus Seed Extract

Citrus seed extract is also sold under many brand names. It is a folk remedy for treating parasites, but there is little hard evidence that this remedy has such an effect. However, some physicians report it is excellent for treating candidiasis. Therefore, for the latter condition, I recommend this product be taken either in capsule, tablet, or in liquid form. Follow the directions on the label.

Activated Charcoal

The ancient Egyptians and Greeks used charcoal as a digestive remedy. It is used for acute stomach and intestinal disorders, food poisoning, drug overdoses, hangovers, and can even be used externally and internally to help relieve gout symptoms. Activated charcoal attracts toxins and bacteria because of its especially large surface area, and helps eliminate them via the intestines. For digestive disorders it is specifically used for intestinal gas and gas pain, abdominal bloating, IBS, and malodorous stools. I have found it helpful in stopping acute flare-ups of Crohn's disease, especially the accompanying sharp, stabbing abdominal pain. Unlike drugs such as simethicone, which disperse gas, activated charcoal reduces gas within the intestine, making it more effective. **However, because it can interfere with the absorption of drugs and nutrients, activated charcoal should not be used for prolonged periods unless directed by a health professional**. Dosage is 2 to 5 tablets or capsules for the first dose, followed by 1 or 2 capsules every half hour. If an acute condition persists for more than 3 days or if you have diarrhea with fever, consult a health professional.

Gamma Oryzanol

Gamma oryzanol is derived from rice bran oil. Research studies have found that it appears to protect the gastrointestinal mucosa and help normalize gastric secretions. In Japanese studies, dosage was between 75 mg to 600 mg per day, with most patients taking 300 mg per day. Improvement was seen in such conditions as anorexia, abdominal pain and distention, eructation, diarrhea, nausea, gastric ulcers, chronic gastritis, and IBS.[4] Results are usually evident within the first 2 to 4 weeks of treatment.

Butyrates

Butyrates are manufactured by intestinal bacteria and are energy sources for the cells that line the colon. With intestinal diseases, butyrates may not be effectively manufactured. Holistic doctors like Jonathan Wright, MD, recommend taking butyrates by enema so that the absorption occurs directly in the colon. In a study of ten patients suffering ulcerative colitis who did not respond to oral or rectal sulfasalazine or prednisone, two weeks' treatment with sodium butyrate resulted in stoppage of bleeding and decrease in stool frequency and inflammation.[5]

Supplements to Be Used with Caution

Iron

While iron is abundant in many of the foods we commonly eat, deficiency of this important mineral is not unusual. This is because our bodies require high levels of iron to function normally. Therefore, if you are iron-deficient, you should supplement with iron. However, supplementation should be undertaken prudently, since excess iron is just as dangerous as too little. Iron overload results in disturbance of the immune system and counters the production of lymphocytes. It can also lead to an iron storage disease known as hemosiderosis.

When taking iron supplements, there are many different forms of iron to choose from. For example, iron ascorbate, aspartate, citrate, gluconate, succinate, and nicconate; ferrous fumarate and sulfate; iron amino acid chelate. You may have to experiment with several products until you find one that is suitable for you. Liquid iron preparations are the most easily tolerated. For all iron supplements, I advise starting at ⅓ or ½ of the recommended dosage, and increase over time. To be safe, after supplementing for a period such as 1 to 2 months, you should have a blood test done to check your iron level.

HCl (Hydrochloric acid)

Hydrochloric acid is a supplement used to increase stomach acidity. Natural food enthusiasts often recommend HCl to persons with digestive problems. HCl is contraindicated unless you have insufficient stomach acidity. Stomach acidity can be monitored by your health professional using the Heidelberg pH capsule or the Gastro Test capsule. If burning or discomfort occurs after taking HCl supplements you should reduce your dosage, as over-supplementation can result in gastritis or even gastric ulcer. Between 1 and 5 capsules are usually taken immediately after eating. In TCM, lack of acid corresponds to a cold condition, therefore a safer alternative is to drink ginger tea with fresh squeezed lime juice before meals.

Chapter Notes

1. Jean Carper, *Food, Your Miracle Medicine* (New York, NY: Harper Collins, 1993) 443.
2. H. Sandberg-Gertzen. "An Open Trial of Cedemin, A Ginkgo Biloba Extract with PAF-Antagonistic Effects for Ulcerative Colitis," *American Journal of Gastroenterology* 88 (1993): 615.
3. A. Belluzzi, C. Brignoli, M.Campieri, A. Pera, S. Boschi, M. Miglioli, "Effects of an Enteric-Coated Fish-Oil Preparation on Relapses of Crohn's Disease," *New England Journal of Medicine* 334 (1996): 1557.

4. S. Kita, "Practical Use of Gamma-Oryzanol on Digestive System Complaints," *Shinyakyto Rinsho* 25.8 (1976): 28.
5. W. Scheppach, H. Sommer, T. Kirchner, G.M. Paganelli, P. Bartram, S. Christi, F. Richter, G. Dusel, H. Kasper, "Effect of Butyrate Enemas on the Colonic Mucosa in Distal Ulcerative Colitis," *Gastroenterology* 103 (1992): 51.

Chapter Four

Symptoms
and Treatments

In this chapter I discuss various digestive conditions that can be treated with different natural methods. Many of the products mentioned under Self Help can be found in health food stores or pharmacies. Products listed under Professional Treatment are available through health professionals, as they are more potent and treat specific syndrome patterns. In undertaking any treatment it is important to be patient in giving these natural remedies time to exert their effects. One should also be mindful that what works for one person may not work for another with the same biomedical condition. This is why health professionals experienced with these remedies and therapies can provide invaluable guidance.

Included under various conditions are case histories, to illustrate the benefits of natural remedies in treating these diseases. For products with their dosages listed, I use the biomedical abbreviations of BID, TID, and QID, which indicate, respectively, twice per day, three times per day, and four times per day.

Adhesions

Adhesions—fibrous bands or scars—can affect the small intestine. They result from prolonged infection or inflammation, or may follow surgery. The scar tissue can disrupt peristalsis, the rhythmic contractions that move partially digested food through the intestine. Spasmodic pain may arise, and the intestine may become obstructed. Exploratory or laparoscopic surgery can remove the adhesions, but recurrence is common. Herbs may be helpful in resolving the scar tissue and obstruction, as well as in regulating intestinal function. However, if you decide to undergo such therapy you should be supervised by a health professional.

Professional Treatment

- Isatis Cooling formula (3 to 4 tablets TID) is especially beneficial for its anti-inflammatory effect, combined with formulas that promote circulation, such as Flavonex (3 tablets TID), or Resinall E (3 tablets TID), which strongly promotes blood circulation. For long-term treatment consider Flavonex (3 to 4 tablets TID) by itself.

Case Study

A 43-year-old woman who had undergone surgery for adhesions of the colon experienced severe abdominal pain and constipation following the procedure. Traditional Chinese diagnosis found that her pulse was sinking and wiry, and her tongue dry. I recommended the formulas Aquilaria 22 (2 tablets TID, increased as necessary) and Flavonex (2 tablets TID) to promote blood circulation. After two weeks she had significantly less pain and constipation.

Anorexia Nervosa and Bulimia

These disorders affect 1 to 2 percent of women between the ages of 12 and 18. About 5 percent of anorexics are male. Holistic doctors believe that zinc deficiency may contribute to these conditions, but psychological considerations are also important. Frequently there is a difficult mother-daughter relationship. In addition to being obsessed with the idea of being fat, there can be great fear in the thought of growing up. About half of anorexics develop bulimia, which is characterized by binge eating followed by purging through induced vomiting, laxatives, diuretics, extreme dieting, or fasting. Bulimics usually have abnormal hunger sensations and then induce vomiting. They also often over-exercise, leading to general depletion of nutrients and energy. Symptoms of anorexia or bulimia can include swollen neck, erosion of the teeth due to excessive vomiting, underweight, weakness, cessation of menstruation, and low pulse rate and blood pressure. Because laxatives deplete the body of potassium, these individuals can also experience irregular heartbeat and even heart failure. Thirty percent of anorexics struggle with the disease all their lives, and the same number experience at least one life-threatening episode.

Self Help

- Withdraw from junk food slowly
- Consider protein powders
- Supplement with multivitamins and minerals such as potassium, selenium, and zinc. Try to get at least 1,800 to 5,600 mg per day of potassium in food or supplement form (consult a food values chart). Take vitamin B_{12} 1,000 to 2,000 mcg per day sublingually (hold the vitamin under your tongue until it is dissolved) to improve mood

- Use acidophilus/bifidus supplements to improve balance of intestinal microflora
- Take herbs such as fennel and ginger to stimulate the appetite

Professional Treatment

- Astra C formula (1 to 2 tablets TID) contains Qi tonic herbs and the readily absorbable zinc citrate
- GB-6 (2 tablets TID; for best results grind the tablets to powder and add to 4 to 8 ounces of hot water) increases circulation in the gastric area, as does Shu Gan (same dosage)
- Use Woman's Balance (2 to 3 tablets TID) to help regulate the menstrual cycle
- Use Astra 18 Diet (3 tablets TID) to promote circulation of Qi
- Use Quiet Digestion (2 tablets TID or 2 tablets with each meal) to promote digestion of food
- For phlegm, use Clear Phlegm (*Wen Dan Tang*) (1 to 2 tablets TID)
- For chronic constipation use the formula Aquilaria 22 (1 to 3 tablets TID)

Case Studies

Case #1

Justine, a fairly healthy looking aerobics instructor in her mid-30s, complained of constipation. She often went on periodic fasts, as encouraged by her spiritual teacher. These fasts would go on for seven days, during which time she consumed only coffee, water, fruit juice, and vegetable broth. Traditional Chinese diagnosis revealed that her pulse was weak and sinking, and tongue normal; she also had dark circles around her eyes, all indicating deficiency of both Qi and kidney yang. She reluctantly complained of shooting abdominal and epigastric pain. I advised her not to go on such extreme fasts for more than twenty-four hours, to adopt a rice and vegetable diet, and to always eat breakfast. I also recommended she take the formulas Gentle Senna (2 tablets TID) and Six Gentlemen (2 tablets TID). After two weeks she reported improvement, but was not willing to eat breakfast due to her hectic schedule. She then canceled her next appointment.

Case #2

Maria, a 24-year-old student, had a ten-year history of bulimia. Her weight fluctuated between 104 and 190 pounds. When she was seen at our clinic she weighed 150 pounds. She was a vegetarian, so to promote her energy level she consumed sugar and sweets. Her pulse was weak and her tongue had a yellow coating. Because she also had PMS, I recommended the formulas Woman's Balance (2 tablets TID) and Astra C (2 tablets TID), as well as a vegetarian protein powder. She was also referred to a hypnotherapist to help improve her self-esteem. After two weeks, she reported more energy than she ever had before.

Appendicitis

Acute appendicitis causes abdominal pain that becomes increasingly severe and localized toward the right lower abdomen. Fever and tenderness usually accompany the pain. Surgery is usually recommended to remove the appendix before it ruptures. Appendicitis that does not require surgery may be treated with herbs.

Professional Treatment

The formulas Isatis Cooling and Coptis Purge Fire (2 tablets of each, 4 to 6 times per day) can be administered.

Case Study

Janice, an administrator at a non-profit organization, was having acute lower quadrant appendicitis-type pain. She was hesitant about going to the hospital since she did not want to undergo surgery. She was counseled to try herbs for twenty-four hours, after which if she was not better to check into the emergency room. She cooked the herbs as a decoction and by the next day, felt 50 percent better. She continued with the herbs and was fully recovered by the second day.

Bacterial Overgrowth

Bacteria can grow in the intestine to the point where absorption of food is impaired. Conventional doctors diagnose this condition only rarely, usually in diabetics and after bowel surgery. Standard medical treatment is to administer antibiotics in a cyclical fashion, such as one week per month. Holistic doctors diagnose this condition more commonly and administer colostrom, acidophilus supplements, and herbal antibiotics.

Professional Treatment

- Acidophilus and bifidus supplements 3 times per day on an empty stomach
- Use Colostroplex (1 to 2 tablets TID) for loose stools (formula has anti-diarrheal and antibacterial effects)
- Use Isatis Gold (2 tablets TID) or Phellostatin (1 to 2 tablets TID): these two herbal formulas are antimicrobial; Phellostatin also protects against deterioration of general health because it contains spleen Qi tonics

• Quiet Digestion (2 tablets TID or 2 tablets with each meal) may also be administered to resolve gas, bloating, and food stagnation

Canker Sores and Cold Sores

Stress, fatigue, or food allergies can trigger canker sores, painful ulcerous sores, usually inside the mouth. Iron deficient anemia, as well as deficiency of vitamins B_1, B_2, B_6, B_{12}, and folic acid, are known to trigger attacks. Severe episodes can lead to fever and swollen glands, and may require antibiotics, antihistamines, or corticosteroid preparations.

Cold sores are caused by the herpes virus, which is usually transmitted by a person who has an active infection. Towels, razors, and eating utensils can spread the herpes virus. Symptoms include fluid-filled blisters, or a red, painful area of the skin. Stress, menstruation, sun exposure, or illness can trigger recurrences. When you have a cold sore, avoid contact with infants as well as those with weak immune systems. If you feel you have a cold sore, consult a physician for an examination and possible tests. Medication, such as acyclovir (Zovirax), may be prescribed.

Self Help

If you have recurrent canker sores, evaluate food sensitivities to citrus fruits, tomatoes, and other high acid level foods. Canker sores may also be caused and aggravated by smoking. Gluten-containing foods such as wheat, rye, oats, barley, and spelt are known to trigger canker sores. To heal active ulcers and sores, take clove oil or myrrh tincture: Dab the liquid on the ulcer several times per day, making sure to hold the liquid in the mouth for as long as possible and moving the tongue to insure that the liquid remains in contact with the ulcer.

- Preparations containing goldenseal, echinacea, and isatis, such as Isatis Gold formula may be used internally, 3 capsules or tablets QID
- Chewable zinc lozenges may be helpful
- Use lemon balm tea by gargling for several minutes and then swallowing the liquid, 3 or more times a day for cold sores
- L-lysine cream may be applied topically for cold sores
- Acidophilus/bifidus, 2 capsules or ½ a teaspoon TID or QID, may be helpful in prevention of and as an adjunct to the above measures
- Consider B-complex and folic acid supplements to prevent canker sores

Professional Treatment

- If a blood test reveals anemia, supplement with a readily absorbable form of iron, such as liquid iron
- Both cold sores and canker sores may be treated with Coptis Purge Fire formula (3 tablets, 4 to 6 times per day); reduce dosage if diarrhea occurs
- For pain, dab Resinall K (½ dropperful, 3 to 6 times per day) on the sore with a cotton swab and hold to the affected area of the mouth for as long as possible (Resinall K contains myrrh and other pain-relieving herbs)
- To prevent canker sores, evaluate for stomach yin deficiency or damp-heat: for stomach yin deficiency, use the formula Clearing (3 tablets TID); for damp-heat, use Isatis Cooling (3 tablets TID) or Phellostatin (2 tablets TID)

• To prevent cold sores, consider the formula Astra Isatis (2 to
  3 tablets TID); with signs of heat combine with Clear Heat
  (2 tablets TID), without heat signs, combine with Power
  Mushrooms (1 to 2 tablets TID)

Case Studies

Case #1

Alicia, a healthy 29-year-old secretary frequently came down
with canker sores, which lasted up to two weeks. Although she
had signs of poor digestion, such as abdominal pain and burning
as well as food intolerance, she was only interested in help for
the canker sores. Traditional Chinese diagnosis found her pulse
slightly fast, and tongue bright red with cracks. As she was currently suffering an outbreak, I suggested that she dab clove oil
on the sore 3 times per day, and take Coptis Purge Fire (3 tablets
QID). She telephoned the next day to say that the canker sores
were gone.

Case #2

Alan, a 35-year-old ulcer patient suffered recurrent cold sores.
Traditional Chinese diagnosis revealed that his pulse was rapid,
and tongue dark red. He also complained of burning and stabbing pains in the epigastrium. I recommended a combination of
Isatis Cooling (3 tablets TID) and Quiet Digestion (2 tablets
TID). I also suggested Coptis Purge Fire (3 tablets QID) specifically for active cold sores. He later reported that after taking the
Isatis Cooling and Quiet Digestion, he experienced fewer inci-
dences of cold sores. He also indicated that the Coptis Purge Fire
reduced the intensity and duration of an outbreak.

Cancers

Colon Cancer

Colon cancer is the second most common cancer in North America. More than 1,200,000 cases are diagnosed each year. Signs and symptoms of colon cancer include rectal bleeding, change in bowel habit, abdominal cramping or pain, blood in the stool (usually microscopic), unexplained anemia, and weight loss. There is an increased risk of colon cancer if there is a family history of colorectal (colon/rectal) cancer, colon polyps, or ulcerative bowel disease.

Non-malignant colon tumors of various types are commonly found in senior citizens. Most, if not all, have the potential to become cancerous, and are therefore surgically removed. Intestinal polyps are considered to be pre-cancerous lesions, and are also customarily removed surgically when discovered. Follow-up exams to check for recurrence are routine. Removal of the colon is usually recommended in cases of familial colonic polyposis and Gardner's syndrome.

Methods for early detection of polyps and tumors include rectal exam, sigmoidoscopy, and stool testing for microscopic blood. Definitive diagnosis is made by X-ray, endoscopy of the colon, and biopsy. Colon cancer is usually treated with surgery, sometimes combined with chemotherapy or radiation therapy.

A high-fat, low fiber diet is the most important contributing lifestyle factor for the development of this cancer. High fat foods, red meat, and alcohol seem to promote development of colon cancer. Fat consumption prompts microorganisms in the colon to make more bile acid, which in turn damages the colon. Heavy drinkers may double or triple their chances of colorectal cancer. Heavy drinking suppresses the immune system, making the body less able to combat the cancer process. Beer appears to be the most, and wine the least, harmful alcoholic beverage; it appears that beer may contain carcinogens such as nitrosamine. Swedish researchers found that brewery workers who drank about seven times as much beer as non-brewery workers had a higher rate of rectal and other forms of cancer.

The most beneficial foods for cancer prevention are those that are high in fiber and seafood. Wheat bran has protective anti-cancer qualities that are not found in oats or corn. Therefore, if you don't have wheat sensitivity you might consider eating home-made wheat bran muffins or bran cereal. Regular consumption of fish may also help prevent polyps and colon cancer. Studies have shown that subjects who took fish oil capsules in large amounts over three months had fewer cancerous cells than subjects who were on a placebo (sugar pill).

Esophageal Tumors

The chief symptoms of esophageal tumors are difficulty in swallowing, unexplained weight loss, regurgitation, and vomiting of blood. Nearly 90 percent of esophageal tumors are malignant. Men are more prone, with heavy smokers and drinkers in their 50s and 60s at highest risk. Surgery and other techniques such as dilation are common modalities of treatment.

Tumors of the Small Intestine

Tumors of the small intestine usually occur between the ages of 40 and 60. The most common symptoms are pain, nausea, vomiting, and bleeding. Weight loss sometimes occurs with malignant tumors. Several types of benign tumors include adenomas, angiomas, leiomyomas, and lipomas. Some benign tumors can cause bleeding, but they do not spread and are not harmful.

Adenocarcinoma, carcinoid tumor, leiomyosarcoma, and lymphoma are examples of malignant tumors. Leiomyosarcoma may cause bleeding, perforation, and obstruction.

Carcinoid tumors grow slowly, and are usually found in the ileum (the lower section of the small intestine) and can spread to the liver, lungs, pancreas, spleen, ovaries, and other organs. These tumors can cause flushing of the skin, diarrhea, and other signs of malabsorption. Diagnosis is usually made through urinalysis.

The standard treatment is to use surgery for benign and malignant tumors when possible. Otherwise, combinations of chemotherapy, radiation, and steroids are used.

Natural Treatment Adjuncts to Conventional Cancer Treatment

The complementary approach to treating digestive and other cancers is to combine nutritional and herbal approaches with the standard medical treatments of surgery, chemotherapy, and radiotherapy. Tobacco, alcohol, artificial sweeteners, preservatives, food additives, pesticides, aluminum, and hydrogenated fats (margarine) should be eliminated; sugar and sweets should be either drastically reduced or completely eliminated. Additionally, chlorinated water should probably be avoided. Most natural practitioners recommend eating a lowfat, high fiber diet based on whole fruits and vegetables. Dairy products are usually restricted, because according to Chinese medicine they are phlegm producing; phlegm causes stagnation of the flow of blood and Qi. Some proponents recommend a vegetarian diet, while others stress the need for adequate protein. From a Chinese medicine standpoint, meat is beneficial, particularly if it is organic and free of hormones, antibiotics, and other chemicals. Exercise to 80 percent capacity is very important, as are visualization, meditation, and the Chinese meditation exercise of Qi Gong, which is widely used in China to treat cancer.

116

+ Beta-carotene (50,000 IU) or mixed carotenoids (30 mg), combined with vitamin A (20,000 IU) daily
+ Vitamin C (1 to 5 g per day; some experts recommend 10 to 20 grams per day; proponents of vitamin C such as Linus Pauling recommend high dosages, whereas other researchers have found that the body is only able to absorb 200 to 250 mg at once)
+ Vitamin E (200 to 800 IU per day)
+ Take B-complex (50 mg of each vitamin) along with folic acid (400 to 800 mcg) daily; some find that B vitamins are too warming in property, and can lead to an increase in symptoms of stress
+ Minerals: basic multimineral (along with iron if you are anemic); use as directed
+ Trace minerals: selenium (200 mcg), zinc (15 to 30 mg), copper (2 to 4 mg), manganese (5 to 20 mg), molybdenum (100 to 1,000 mcg) daily
+ Use flax oil (1 to 3 tablespoons) or ground flax seed (1 to 3 tablespoons) daily
+ *L. acidophilus* helps suppress the enzyme activity that converts otherwise harmless substances into cancer-causing chemicals in the colon. According to a study conducted at the New England Medical Center, acidophilus milk caused dangerous enzyme activity to drop between 40 to 80 percent[1]

Professional Treatment

+ Colonics and coffee enemas are sometimes recommended
+ Shiitake mushrooms can be incorporated as part of the diet several times per week for immune support
+ Proteolytic enzymes can be considered
+ Herbs (Essiac, hoxsey, Chinese anti-cancer and tonic herbs) administered by an experienced herbalist

- Astra Essence formula (3 tablets TID), as a general tonic, helps strengthen the body
- Marrow Plus (3 to 4 tablets TID) promotes production of red and white blood cells that are destroyed by conventional therapies
- Use Regeneration (2 to 3 tablets TID) for long-term maintenance. Designed by master herbalist Dr. Fung Fung, Regeneration is a combination of special anti-toxin, tonifying, and circulation promoting herbs
- Colostroplex (1 to 2 tablets TID) can be taken when diarrhea is present
- Isatis Cooling (3 tablets TID) is helpful for burning abdominal cramping and heat signs
- Quiet Digestion (2 tablets QID or as needed) is used for nausea and abdominal discomfort, common side effects of cancer treatment
- For weight loss, especially accompanied by diarrhea, use Source Qi formula (3 to 5 tablets TID)
- Use Power Mushrooms formula (2 tablets TID) which contains ganoderma, tremella and poria, to boost the immune system
- Bovine and shark cartilages have been used as an experimental cancer treatment. Shark cartilage must be taken at a dosage of 60 to 80 mg per day and bovine cartilage at 9 g per day, in order to be effective
- Magnet therapy (see a professional for explanation of effects)

Case Studies

Case #1

Alma, an African American in her late 60s, came in with her daughter and grandson, which I thought was a good sign since many cultures believe in family support during appointments with professionals. Alma's colon had been removed due to cancer, and she wore a colostomy bag. Her symptoms were weakness and feeling cold all the time. Traditional Chinese diagnosis revealed that her pulse was sinking and slow, and tongue pale and dry. The treatment strategy was to invigorate blood circulation in order to help the body heal from surgery, and to support Qi and blood due to weakened state. She was advised to take Source Qi (3 tablets TID) and Shen Gem (3 tablets TID) formulas, first in tea form (tablets were ground into a powder and then steeped in hot water), and after three weeks she was switched to tablets. Following two months of herbal therapy, she reported her digestion was better and that she felt much stronger.

Case #2

Doug, 44, had developed intense abdominal burning, nausea, and insomnia following chemotherapy treatments for colorectal cancer. Traditional Chinese diagnosis found that his pulse was flooding, and tongue red. I recommended Isatis Cooling (5 tablets TID) with Quiet Digestion (1 to 2 tablets as needed) for nausea. Within two weeks he said the burning was reduced by 50 percent. He also said that when he was awakened at night by abdominal burning, he would take the Isatis Cooling (3 tablets), which provided relief. As he was doing well on the protocol, the same herbs were continued for another month. At this point, the abdominal burning was being controlled by the Isatis Cooling and he was no longer experiencing nausea. His pulse had slowed, his tongue was now pale with redness around the edges. I then recommended reducing the dosage of Isatis Cooling (3 tablets TID) and adding Six Gentlemen (3 tablets TID) formula to tonify spleen Qi and reduce cramping. Over the next few months he did so well that he took the Isatis Cooling only on an as-needed basis, a few times a week, and continued a maintenance dosage of Six Gentlemen (3 tablets TID).

Case #3

Blair, 65, had undergone chemotherapy for lymphoma. He was suffering from severe constipation, intestinal gas, poor appetite, night sweats, fatigue, and dry cough. Traditional Chinese diagnosis revealed that his pulse was sinking, and tongue dry. Tremella and American Ginseng formula (5 tablets TID) was given to reduce night sweats and treat the dry cough. Gentle Senna (3 tablets TID) was recommended for the constipation. After two weeks he reported that all symptoms had improved. Over the next few months, Tremella and American Ginseng was withdrawn and replaced with Shen Gem (3 tablets TID), which tonifies Qi and blood.

Case #4

Thelma, 43, developed low red and white blood cell counts following chemo- and radiotherapy for breast cancer. Other symptoms included nausea, fatigue, and abdominal cramping following chemotherapy. Traditional Chinese diagnosis found that her pulse was sinking and thin, and tongue pale and dry. Thelma was advised to take Quiet Digestion (2 tablets as needed) a few days to one week following each session of chemotherapy for the nausea and cramping. Once her digestion was restored, she took Marrow Plus (3 tablets TID), which boosted her blood cell counts; Backbone (3 tablets TID) was also recommended, to tonify the kidney and strengthen the effects of Marrow Plus. Thelma's medical doctors were impressed with her improved blood counts. She was then able to continue with her chemotherapy treatments as scheduled. After three months of herbal therapy, her blood counts were within the normal range.

Candidiasis

According to holistic professionals, *Candida* yeast infection can cause or contribute to all digestive symptoms, and can induce other symptoms such as fatigue, headaches, joint and muscle aches, and menstrual irregularities. Western doctors, on the other hand, feel that candidiasis is only a problem with vaginal yeast infection, thrush, and *Candida* esophagitis.

Normally, healthy intestinal bacteria, the right acid/alkaline balance, and a properly working immune system keep *Candida,* a resident member of our intestinal tract, from getting out of control. However, immune suppressive drugs such as antibiotics, hormones (including birth control pills), steroids, and chemotherapy can result in yeast overgrowth.

I have found that an anti-yeast diet, as well as dietary supplements and herbs, are very useful in treating digestive disorders. This is especially true if there is a past history of using the above-mentioned drugs (particularly antibiotics), and if there are such accompanying signs as a history of vaginal yeast infections, athlete's foot, jock itch, or fungal infections of the nails or skin. Other indications include symptoms that worsen in damp weather or in moldy buildings, and cravings for sweets and yeast-containing foods (such as beer, wine, bread, and cheese). Although physicians can administer tests to determine if you have excess levels of *Candida,* such tests are often expensive. Furthermore, it is possible to have a sensitivity to normal levels of yeast.

The Digestive Clearing program described in Chapter Five consists of a diet that is free of alcohol, sweets, and yeast-containing foods.

Self Help

- Pau D'Arco tea (6 cups daily) has anti-*Candida* properties and is an excellent beverage for those undergoing anti-*Candida* therapy
- Garlic has antifungal properties, but should not be used by persons with hot constitutions or with a sensitivity to garlic (dosage is 1 or 2 cloves per day)
- Yeast Guard is a homeopathic suppository that can be used
- Citrus seed extract (use as directed) can be considered

Professional Treatment

- Phellostatin is a formula I helped develop and is designed to alter the ecology of the intestines; the formula contains anti-yeast herbs along with digestive tonics. General dosage is 1 tablet TID for the first two weeks, and 2 to 3 tablets TID thereafter. The therapies listed below may be useful in conjunction, to either assist the digestive system or to promote rapid elimination of yeast. By using several natural therapies simultaneously it is possible to achieve comparable results to prescription drugs
- Biocidin (use as directed) helps to rapidly kill off yeast; it should not be used without Phellostatin or a digestive tonic such as Six Gentlemen because it is very cold in property, and Phellostatin and Six Gentlemen can offset Biocidin's coldness
- Aquilaria 22 (1 to 3 tablets TID) can be used alone or with Phellostatin in cases of constipation; it has anti-yeast and anti-parasitic properties
- Colostroplex (bovine colostrum) (1 to 2 tablets TID; reduce dosage if constipation occurs) is used with Phellostatin to

improve digestive immunity and to treat diarrhea. Colostroplex has anti-viral and antibacterial properties and may have anti-fungal properties as well

- Quiet Digestion (2 tablets TID) treats food stagnation and acute digestive symptoms
- Vagistatin (1 to 2 capsules at bedtime) is an herbal antifungal vaginal suppository

Prescription Antifungal Medications

- **Nystatin** is an antifungal medication that is over forty years old. It comes in cream, ointment, suppository, tablet, and powder forms. The advantage of the powder form is that it can be used in a gargle, douche, or enema for rapid effect. Nystatin is safe for long-term usage, but follow your physician's dosage recommendations carefully. Symptoms may temporarily worsen when starting any antifungal medication—this is known as a die-off reaction. Rebound reactions, in which the yeast infection recurs with severe intensity when the drug is discontinued, also occur, which is why I recommend that Phellostatin herbal formula be taken with these drugs
- **Nizoral (ketoconazole)** is a broad-spectrum antifungal drug. Some patients are better able to tolerate Nizoral than Nystatin; however, a small percentage experience liver problems from use of this drug. If you have a history of liver problems, or if you take this drug for over three months, your liver function should be monitored. Since Nizoral is toxic to the liver, I suggest that Ecliptex herbal formula (2 tablets TID) or milk thistle (follow label directions) be taken two weeks for every week on Nizoral
- **Diflucan (fluconazole)** is more effective than Nizoral at combating yeast infections. It works over a shorter period of

time and is not harmful to the liver. Unfortunately, Diflucan is expensive, at over $10 per pill, whereas Nizoral costs about $1 to $2 per pill

- **Sporanox (itraconazole)** appears to be more effective than Nizoral. Some patients may be intolerant to Diflucan, but are better able to tolerate Sporanox and vice versa

Case Studies

Case #1

A woman in her late 30s came to be treated for PMS, sudden weight gain, fatigue, and abdominal cramping. Her medical doctor, whose diagnosis was *Candida*-related complex, had previously treated her with Diflucan. The client reported that the Diflucan therapy had lessened her fatigue and depression by about 50 percent. I suggested that she follow an anti-*Candida* diet, and also recommended she take the formula Woman's Balance (2 tablets QID) for the PMS, as well as Unlocking (2 tablets QID) for the abdominal cramping. With this protocol, she noticed a definite improvement of her symptoms in three months.

Case #2

Emelio, a 45-year-old cook, had numerous health complaints including sinusitis, frequent ear infections, chronic sore throat, frequent and burning urination, fatigue, low back pain, poor sleep, joint pain, tinnitus, hypertension, poor digestion, constipation, and chronic cold hands and feet. He had a history of hepatitis and had been recently diagnosed as having chronic fatigue syndrome by a holistic medical doctor who placed Emelio on antifungal drugs, including Nystatin and Diflucan. He had also prescribed acupuncture, vitamins, and homeopathics. Even though all these remedies had helped, Emelio reported he was so tired he could "barely make it through the day," and that he still had the abovementioned complaints.

Traditional Chinese diagnosis found that his pulse was racing, and tongue purplish, with a thick coating on the sides. He had signs of heat in the Upper Burner and kidney yang deficiency, therefore the treatment principle was to tonify the yang and remove pathogenic heat and dampness. We recommended that he abstain from alcohol, reduce his intake of sugar, including fruit sugar, and increase his protein intake. Since he admitted to ejaculating several times a day, he was urged to limit this, because ejaculation is said to deplete the kidney Essence, causing fatigue, low back pain, weak knees, and frequent urination. He was advised to take Coptis Purge Fire (3 tablets QID) with Astra Isatis (3 tablets QID). During his next visit two weeks later, he reported slightly more energy and less burning with urination. As his pulse was not as excessive, and his face less red, the dosage of Coptis Purge Fire

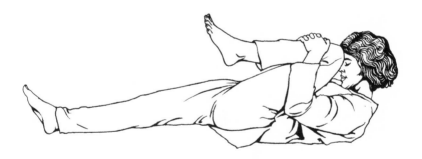

Wind Eliminating Posture
This position relieves intestinal gas. Lie on your back and relax as you breathe. Bend your right knee and wrap your arms around the leg pulling it toward your chest. Raise your head, bringing your forehead to your knee. Hold for 3 to 5 seconds. Lower your leg and head to the floor and relax. Repeat with your left leg, then repeat with both legs simultaneously. This exercise should be performed at least 10 times.

was reduced (2 tablets QID), and Shen Gem (2 tablets QID) was added, while the dosage of Astra Isatis remained the same.

After one month on the second protocol, Emelio reported feeling more energy and no longer had burning with urination. His pulse was hollow and slightly irregular, but his tongue, however, was normal. At this point, Coptis Purge Fire was discontinued, but because fatigue was still a problem, Power Mushrooms was recommended. The new regimen thus consisted of Power Mushrooms (2 tablets QID), Astra Isatis (2 tablets QID), and Shen Gem (2 tablets QID). Emelio noticed some digestive discomfort after starting this protocol and was instructed to reduce the dosage of Power Mushrooms. But he then indicated that he had experienced an increase in energy after starting on the Power Mushrooms, he thus elected to stay on the original dosage. Although his treatment protocol varied over the next nine months, most of Emelio's symptoms disappeared through continued herbal therapy.

Case #3

Eleanor, a graphic designer in her early 40s, complained of severe PMS, weight gain, chronic fatigue, fibromyalgia, and depression. A battery of tests at Stanford University were inconclusive. She visited an MD specializing in chronic fatigue syndrome, who placed her on a trial therapy of the antifungal medication Diflucan, which appeared to improve her symptoms by about 50 percent. She sought additional relief at our clinic.

Eleanor's initial traditional Chinese syndrome pattern was one of damp-heat, primarily of dampness, which was manifested by symptoms of overweight and worsening of joint and muscle pain in rainy weather or damp environments. Her pulse was slippery, and tongue had a grayish yellow coating. Based on her pattern presentation and the fact that she was benefiting from the Diflucan, and that she had been on several courses of antibiotics each year during the past decade to treat cystitis and bronchial infections—additional indicators of damp-heat—we decided to start her on an anti-*Candida* diet that eliminated alcohol, sweets, and yeast-containing foods. We also suggested two herbal formulas, Phellostatin (1 tablet TID the first week, 2 TID tablets thereafter) and Woman's Balance (2 tablets TID), as well as Astra Diet Tea, to be consumed several times throughout the day as a substitute for sweets, and to promote energy and reduce phlegm.

Eleanor had great trouble adhering to the recommended diet, so it was not surprising that after three weeks she had noticed little change in her symptoms. We encouraged her to do her best, stressing that if she stopped her nightly wine consumption she would in all likelihood feel better and even lose weight. Nevertheless, she did notice less fluid retention during her first premenstrual phase (since coming to our clinic), but the mood swings and irritability remained. Six weeks after starting the herbal formulas and following the diet as best as she could, she finally reduced her wine intake to Saturday nights only. She had also lost 5 pounds and felt more clear headed. During her second premenstrual phase, she noticed significantly fewer mood swings, less irritability, and less fluid retention. By her third period, nearly all PMS symptoms were resolved. At this time, we recommended that she stay on the Woman's Balance premenstrually, and take Phellostatin (same dosage) and Aspiration (3 tablets TID). The latter was used to relieve depression as it contains specific herbs such as vervain, polygala (*yuan zhi*), and albizzia (*he huan pi*) for that purpose.

Case #4

William, a 30-year-old sales representative, complained of fatigue, athlete's foot, and chronic intestinal gas. He was away from home 2 to 3 weeks every month, and undoubtedly his constant restaurant eating was a major contributing factor to his digestive disorders.

In addition, after his daily meetings and sales calls, he usually had several alcoholic beverages; and when he was home, he typically smoked marijuana to relax. Traditional Chinese diagnosis revealed that his pulse was slow, sinking and slightly wiry, and his tongue red with a thick, greasy yellow coating. I recommended Phello-statin (2 tablets TID) to tonify the spleen, clear heat, and rid the body of fungus. He was also given Quiet Digestion (2 tablets TID), since it possesses herbs that address flatulence, resolve dampness, and relieve food stagnation, which causes intestinal gas. I also suggested 2 capsules of PB 8 acidophilus to be taken at bedtime.

In terms of dietary and lifestyle habits, he was advised to reduce or eliminate alcohol, which promotes growth of yeast, and to reduce or stop his marijuana use, which through its laxative effects will over time weaken the spleen and lead to accumulation of dampness. Furthermore, fungal mold is known to contaminate marijuana. I also recommended low sugar and non-fermented foods, and gave him a supplemental list of foods that can cause gas such as beans, peas, wheat, oats, bran, brussels sprouts, cabbage, corn, rutabaga, and dairy products.

At his next visit one month later, William reported that the symptoms of gas were reduced by about 50 percent and that his energy level had increased slightly. But he also expressed his disappointment that his condition was not cured. His pulse was thin and wiry, and although his tongue no longer had a thick coating, it was now pale in the center and red on the edges. I asked him if he had made any of the recommended dietary and lifestyle changes, to which he replied that because he traveled so often, it was difficult—if not impossible—to change his habits while on the road. I pointed out that if he wanted to "cure" his intestinal gas he would have to make the dietary changes, and suggested that he locate health food stores and perhaps restaurants that serve healthy cuisines in the cities he visited instead of going to standard restaurants. I also indicated that he should get more exercise.

With regard to his herbal therapy, I recommended that he finish the bottle of Phellostatin that he had (2 tablets TID), remain on Quiet Digestion (2 tablets as needed) and PB 8 (2 capsules at bedtime), and to add Ecliptex (2 tablets TID) to soothe the liver.

By his next visit a month later he had reduced his alcohol intake to one drink per night. He indicated that the problem with gas remained about the same, but Quiet Digestion proved symptomatically effective. He also reported that he had developed insomnia and acid reflux, which he first tried to blame on his reduction in alcohol, but later admitted he was having marital problems, largely as a result of being away from home so long. William's pulse remained wiry and his tongue unchanged. At this point, I added Ease Plus (2 tablets QID) to his treatment plan, in order to calm the nerves, spread liver Qi, and reduce stomach acidity. Quiet Digestion and PB 8 were continued at the same dosages.

Discussion: The herbs appeared to be helpful, but did not resolve William's condition. This was because of his excessive traveling, in addition to marital problems, both of which created stress such that he relied on alcohol for relief.

Candida Esophagitis

This is an infection of the esophagus caused by *Candida* yeast, and usually occurs in people with depressed immune systems. Symptoms include inflammation of the esophagus, with painful swallowing. Conventional treatment is to use antifungal drugs, such as Nizoral. Concurrent herbal therapy can be undertaken by combining Phellostatin (2 to 3 tablets TID) and herbal antifungals such as Pau D'Arco tea (8 cups per day) and Biocidin (1 to 6 drops with meals).

Case Study

Carl, 38, was undergoing chemotherapy and developed *Candida* esophagitis and thrush, causing difficulty swallowing. He was being treated with Nizoral. Traditional Chinese diagnosis showed that he had a heavy yellow tongue coating and his pulse was sinking and rapid. I recommended Pau D'Arco tea (8 cups per day), Biocidin (3 drops in water, gargled before each meal), and Phellostatin (3 tablets TID before meals). After one week the thrush was significantly reduced and he was having an easier time swallowing. His tongue coating was also not as thick.

Chronic Constipation

Constipation is difficult to define. Conventional medical texts say that it is not necessary to have a bowel movement every day, and suggest that having only three bowel movements a week falls within the normal range. Herbalists, on the other hand, point out that the physiology of the gastrointestinal tract is such that one to three movements per day should be the norm. Specifically, each meal that enters the stomach triggers reflex movements in the colon, and can lead to a bowel movement. Other factors, such as fat in the diet, stress, and inactivity during the daylight hours may slow the process, but it is normal to have at least one bowel movement a day upon rising in the morning or following the morning meal. Constipation that comes on suddenly or persists may require a visit to the doctor to rule out causes such as intestinal obstruction, hypothyroidism, or side effects from medication.

If you do not have regular bowel movements, it is important *not* to resort to laxatives to solve the problem. In fact, laxatives — both chemical and herbal — are a common cause of chronic constipation. While they can be used occasionally, habitual use creates dependence, and not only damages the bowel, but upsets the body's mineral balance. Finally, when discontinuing laxatives, do so slowly, rather than stopping "cold turkey," so that your digestive system has a chance to readjust.

Chronic Bad Breath

A 55-year-old woman complained of chronic bad breath, belching and loose stools, a metallic (bitter) taste in her mouth, and work related stress. She was also ten pounds overweight. Traditional Chinese diagnosis revealed that her pulse was wiry, and tongue red with a yellow coating. She was advised to take the formula Clearing (3 tablets TID). After one month there was no significant change, so she was switched to Colostroplex (1 tablet TID), which seemed to help the stools become more formed. Because she still had belching, Woman's Balance (3 tablets TID) was suggested. After two months the belching was relieved, but the bad breath and metallic taste in the mouth persisted. Since bad breath and other symptoms such as hers usually respond to herbs within a month, and the fact she had rheumatic fever as a child and had been on penicillin from ages thirteen to nineteen, I suspected that she might have undiagnosed candidiasis, and thus recommended anti-*Candida* therapy. It was suggested that she eliminate all sugars, including fruit, for two weeks, as well as yeast-containing foods. She was not an alcohol drinker. Phellostatin formula was then introduced, and Clearing stopped. Thus, her protocol was Phellostatin (2 tablets TID), Colostroplex (1 tablet TID), and Woman's Balance (2 tablets TID). Although the herbal regimen was somewhat involved because of all the formulas she was taking, it seemed to be the only treatment that improved her breath.

Self Help

- Eat more fiber. Fiber increases the bulk of the stool and binds water, thus making a softer stool. The best sources of fiber are fresh fruits and vegetables. Incorporate psyllium products or soluble fiber, such as oat bran and guar gum, which are easily digested, into your diet
- Set aside a specific time each day (usually after breakfast or dinner) for having a bowel movement
- Do not resist the urge to have a bowel movement
- Exercise daily
- Do not use enemas regularly
- Drink eight glasses of warm or hot water daily; according to Chinese medicine warm or hot water relaxes the intestines

Professional Treatment

- For occasional constipation, in addition to suggestions listed above, use Gentle Senna (2 to 3 tablets TID)
- For severe constipation, or constipation due to antibiotic use, consider the formulas Aquilaria 22 (2 to 3 tablets TID) along with Gentle Senna (1 to 2 tablets TID); and acidophilus/bifidus products (use as directed)
- For constipation in the weak and seniors, use Eight Treasures (2 tablets TID) along with Aquilaria 22 (1 to 3 tablets TID)

Case Studies

Case #1

A chiropractor with a ten-year history of constipation, despite incorporating a fiber-rich diet and psyllium products into her regimen, started using 2 tablets TID of Aquilaria 22. After one week the dosage was increased to 3 tablets TID. After another week, she began to have regular bowel movements.

Case #2

A 51-year-old woman came into our clinic with a conventional diagnosis of IBS. Her main complaint was chronic constipation, which was only relieved by drinking senna tea. She reported that all kinds of food gave her indigestion, which started as a burning in the throat and then turned into nausea and bloating twenty minutes after eating. She also complained of insomnia, which was relieved somewhat with Elavil, the dosage of which had just recently been increased. Traditional Chinese diagnosis revealed that her pulse was wiry, and tongue normal-colored and dry. She also appeared to be a worrier. I gave an herbal tea based on Calm Spirit and Woman's Balance and told her to take Quiet Digestion before each meal. Dietary recommendations involved avoiding fruit (which can ferment in the stomach, causing bloating) for one week, exercising (light aerobics), and going for a walk after each meal. After reading about the side effects of Elavil (including indigestion and constipation), she became concerned and began reducing the dosage under the direction of her doctor over a period of three months, while incorporating the herbs. Under this regimen, all symptoms gradually improved.

Case #3

A woman in her 30s, with a ten-year history of heroin abuse, suffered from chronic constipation, which was only relieved by senna tea and enemas. She wanted to take herbs that were more balancing. She was already on a high fiber diet and was instructed to increase her water intake to six to eight glasses of hot water a day. She was advised to take Aquilaria 22 (3 tablets TID) and acidophilus (2 capsules per day). After three weeks there was no change in her bowel movements. She was then instructed to increase Aquilaria 22 to 5 tablets TID. After six weeks there was still no change, so I recommended the liver formula Ecliptex (2 tablets TID) to move liver Qi; she discontinued acidophilus, but maintained the Aquilaria 22. Four weeks later she began having regular bowel movements without the senna tea.

Case #4

Kayla, 40, underwent "spring cleanses" each year for the past ten years. The cleanses consisted of daily enemas for a week, followed by modified fasts. In addition, she took colonics approximately four times a year. Despite looking fairly energetic, there were deep, dark circles around her eyes. Her main problems were constipation, overweight, and PMS. She took herbal laxatives on a daily basis. Traditional Chinese diagnosis found that her pulse was slow and deep, and her tongue pale and dry.

I counseled her against the regular colonics and enemas, except for periods of extreme constipation, because such practices were draining her overall energy. An examination of her diet revealed insufficient fiber intake. For breakfast, she usually ate nothing, or went out with friends for eggs, potatoes, and toast. For lunch she would have a bowl of soup, and for dinner, a salad. She may have also indulged in junk food, as she was 15 to 20 pounds overweight (her weight problem was not due to hormonal dysfunction). I suggested she eat a breakfast of cereal with prunes each morning, and a more substantial lunch, perhaps salad or soup and maybe a vegetarian sandwich (she was a vegetarian). For dinner, we agreed that she would have some protein, rice, and a cooked vegetable. I also advised fruit for snacks and drinking hot water, with some lemon if she wished. In terms of herbal remedies, I recommended Gentle Senna (2 tablets TID) and Eight Treasures (2 tablets TID). Within two weeks, she reported greater regularity.

Crohn's Disease and Ulcerative Colitis

Crohn's disease and ulcerative colitis are classifications of inflammatory bowel disease (IBD). They are similar conditions, however ulcerative colitis occurs in the colon and the rectum, while Crohn's disease, also called regional enteritis, affects any segment of the alimentary canal, from the mouth to the anus. More commonly Crohn's disease involves the last part of the small intestine, called the ileum. Mild cases of both diseases can cause such symptoms as intestinal cramping and diarrhea. Severe cases can involve bloody diarrhea, bowel obstruction, fever, weight loss, and in the case of Crohn's disease, joint pain, and inflammation in other areas of the body. Diagnosis of either condition is confirmed by barium X-rays, colonoscopy, and biopsy. Conventional treatment consists of medications, including antibiotics and immunosuppressive drugs, as well as corticosteroids, asulfazine, ascol, metronidazole (Flagyl), and chemotherapy drugs. Surgery may be required for bowel obstruction or chronic abscesses, but rates of recurrence after surgery are high.

Either form of inflammatory bowel disease is associated with an increased risk of colon cancer. Parasitic infections can mimic IBD, and I believe those with IBD are more prone to contracting such infections. If parasites are either the cause or a complication, they must be treated first (see "Parasites," later in this chapter).

Crohn's Disease and Food

At the Addenbrookes Hospital, in Cambridge, England, British doctors have been successfully treating active Crohn's disease by determining which foods trigger a flare-up, and then eliminating them from the diet. According to Dr. John O. Hunter, this regimen has worked just as well as surgery and drugs: "Patients who develop a satisfactory diet have overall relapse rates of less

135

than ten per year, which matches the success of surgery." According to Dr. Hunter, "Diet is more successful than medication. Foods most likely to induce flare-ups are wheat, dairy products, cruciferous vegetables, corn, yeast, tomatoes, citrus fruits, and eggs."[2] There may also be a link between flare-ups and frequent eating of cereal and excessive sweets.

Professional Treatments

- The formulas Isatis Cooling (3 to 5 tablets TID) and Colostroplex (1 to 3 tablets TID) have been used with success along with Quiet Digestion (1 to 2 tablets with each meal) to help assimilate food
- For stabbing pain and inflammation, use Isatis Cooling alone
- For diarrhea, use Source Qi (3 to 5 tablets TID) combined with Colostroplex (1 to 3 tablets TID)
- For diarrhea and inflammation, use Phellostatin (1 to 3 tablets TID) with Colostroplex, or Isatis Cooling with Colostroplex
- For bloody stools, administer Formula H (3 to 5 tablets TID) and Colostroplex (1 to 3 tablets TID)
- Six Gentlemen (3 tablets TID) and Astra Essence (3 tablets TID) are good follow-up formulas for tonifying and strengthening the body

Case Studies

Case #1
Eloise, a 30-year-old female with a five-year history of Crohn's disease, suddenly developed rectal bleeding and mucous, and up to twenty bowel movements per day. She had alternating diarrhea and small stools, along with constant, severe cramping, and alternating fever and chills. As she had already had a portion of her intestine removed, the next step she faced was a colostomy.

She was taking 50 mg per day of prednisone plus Asacol (mesalamine). Traditional Chinese diagnosis found her pulse was sinking and rapid and her tongue had a thick, greasy yellow coating. I recommended Formula H (3 tablets TID) along with Colostroplex (1 tablet TID), for the first week. I also counseled her to adjust her diet to consist mostly of soups, rice, and lean protein. As there was little change in her symptoms after two weeks, I recommended the dosages of both formulas be increased—Formula H to 5 tablets TID, and Colostroplex to 2 tablets TID. I also suggested she start on Quiet Digestion (1 tablet before and after each meal). The first few days on this revised regimen, her symptoms worsened, but by the end of the second week she experienced a reduction in bowel movements, to about ten per day. She also had more energy and less cramping. She continued the aforementioned protocol for another four weeks, at which time she was having six bowel movements per day; her episodes of fever were now infrequent, and intestinal cramping markedly diminished. She had reduced the Prednisone to 20 mg per day. Her pulse was sinking and had slowed down. Her tongue was pale and the coating was thinner. At this point I recommended she start on Isatis Cooling (3 tablets TID) and reduce the dosage of Formula H (3 tablets TID). She continued with Colostroplex at the same dosage (2 tablets TID).

She stayed on this protocol for another month, at which time her energy had increased dramatically as well as her mental outlook. Her gastroenterologist was willing to delay the surgery. The blood and mucous in her stools were now infrequent and the intestinal cramping now occurred only about once a day. To resolve the cramping, she usually took an extra dosage of Isatis Cooling (3 tablets) along with the 3 to 9 tablets that were recommended per day. She had also reduced the Prednisone to 10 mg per day. Her pulse was now sinking and had a normal rate, and her tongue coating was almost normal.

At this juncture, I advised that she eliminate Formula H and substitute Phellostatin (2 tablets TID), which has tonic herbs as well as heat-clearing and antifungal herbs. She remained on Isatis Cooling (3 tablets TID and as needed) as well as Colostroplex (2 tablets TID). Over the next six months she was able to return to work part-time, as the fatigue and bloody and mucosal stools were all completely resolved. She had also stopped the Prednisone but continued to take Asacol. As of this writing, in addition to the daily herbal formulas, consisting of Six Gentlemen (3 tablets TID) and Colostroplex (1 tablet TID), she also takes Isatis Cooling (3 tablets as needed), practices yoga, and participates in counseling.

Case #2

A 28-year-old woman with ulcerative colitis initially came in with chronic fatigue and diarrhea, which were controlled after she started on a combination of Source Qi (4 tablets TID) and Quiet Digestion (2 tablets TID). She maintained this protocol for six months, after which her main symptoms were cramping and mucous in the stools. Laboratory tests revealed excessive amounts of bacteria in her stools. I recommended that she continue with the Source Qi formula and also start on Isatis Cooling (2 tablets TID), which has antibacterial, phlegm (mucous) resolving, and blood circulating properties. She was counseled on diet as well as on developing a mission statement and a daily stress reduction plan. She was also advised to start acidophilus and bifidus supplementation. After thirty days, she no longer experienced cramping or mucous in the stools. I then recommended she stop Isatis Cooling, but continue with Source Qi, Quiet Digestion, and acidophilus and bifidus.

Case #3

A woman in her early 40s, with a high stress job and a biomedical diagnosis of ulcerative colitis with severe rectal bleeding, was put on a rectal suppository called Rowasa (mesalamine). Being an herbalist, she was reluctant to take this drug and therefore discontinued its use. Her attempt at self-treatment with herbs was unsuccessful and two weeks later the bleeding returned. I suggested that she use Rowasa every two to three days instead of daily, and start on Formula H (5 tablets TID) along with Colostroplex (2 tablets per day). Within a month she reported good results with using the suppository every three days and taking the herbs every day. I believe that in time she should be able to be weaned off the suppository completely.

Case #4

Rod, a psychologist in his mid-30s, had his ileum removed more than ten years ago due to severe ulcerative colitis. Since then, every few months he had episodes of severe diarrhea and dehydration that forced him to be hospitalized. When we first saw him at our clinic, he was having phantom pain and tenesmus, tiredness, and joint pain, which was particularly severe during changes in weather. Despite wearing a colostomy bag, he lived an active life and could not trace his flare-ups to any specific stressor. Traditional Chinese diagnosis showed that his pulse was fast and wiry, his tongue swollen, red, and cracked. My recommendation was to take 3 tablets TID of Formula H and increase to 5 tablets TID over a three week period. I also suggested Colostroplex (2 tablets BID). After three weeks he reported less tenesmus, fatigue, and pain. He also felt his joint pain had improved. He remained on this protocol for another month, at which time his pulse was thin and had slowed down considerably, and his tongue was normal. I then recommended he start on Six Gentlemen (3 tablets TID) to tonify his digestive system and for him to decrease the Colostroplex (1 tablet BID).

Diabetic Intestinal Disorders

Chronic diabetes causes various forms of neuropathy, a degeneration of the nerves. Diabetic neuropathy can affect the entire digestive tract. When the nerves of the stomach are involved, the condition is known as diabetic gastroparesis, a partial or incomplete paralysis of the stomach muscles. The emptying of the stomach becomes erratic due to partial paralysis of the intestinal and sphincter muscles. Vomiting of fluid and partially digested food is the main symptom. The most common medical treatment is administration of a drug called Metoclopramide, which stimulates gastric emptying and allays nausea. This drug is not effective for all patients.

When the intestinal nerves are involved, diarrhea or fecal incontinence is likely to occur because of impairment of both sensation and function of the anal sphincter. Malabsorption can result from bacterial overgrowth, non-tropical sprue, or pancreatic insufficiency. Antibiotics are often administered on a cyclical basis to control diarrhea due to bacterial overgrowth.

Professional Treatment

From a Chinese medicine perspective, treatment is based on the patient's constitution and symptoms, which in these conditions indicate that the body's energy is not in harmony.

- An herbal approach for diarrhea is to use Colostroplex (1 to 3 tablets TID) and acidophilus and FOS to control bacterial overgrowth, possibly in addition to herbal formulas with antibiotic properties, such as Astra Isatis (2 tablets TID), which also tonify the body
- Use Quiet Digestion (2 tablets TID or with each meal) to help the digestive system break down food more efficiently

- Pancreatic enzymes (use as directed) may be administered to improve pancreatic function
- Nerve damage is usually treated by using a kidney tonic, such as Astra Essence (3 tablets TID) and Flavonex (3 tablets TID), which has herbs to improve blood circulation
- Diabetes depletes fluids according to Chinese medicine, therefore Yin-nourishing formulas, such as Nine Flavor Tea (3 tablets TID) and Clearing (3 tablets TID), may be useful

Diarrhea

Diarrhea is characterized by the frequent passage of watery stools. Some of the more common causes are viruses, food poisoning, parasites such as *Giardia,* anxiety and nervousness, or reactions to food, alcohol, or medications. Antibiotics, antacids, and other products containing magnesium, antihypertensives, laxatives that are not bulk forming, and medications for irregular heartbeat can all cause diarrhea.

Because diarrhea is a healthy eliminative function that is intended to rid the gut of the irritant causing the problem, experts consider it best to let diarrhea run its course if possible, while using rehydration products to prevent dehydration. Seek medical assistance when severe diarrhea renders you weak, when your temperature is above 101°F (38.3°C), when there is blood or black tarry stools, or when the diarrhea persists for more than ten days. Other symptoms accompanying diarrhea that warrant medical attention include severe abdominal pain, confusion, unresponsiveness, or dizziness while standing.

One type of frequently occurring diarrhea that deserves a few more words here is that due to antibiotic use. Antibiotics can cause the intestines to become inflamed. The result is diarrhea, abdominal cramps, and fever. The symptoms usually begin four

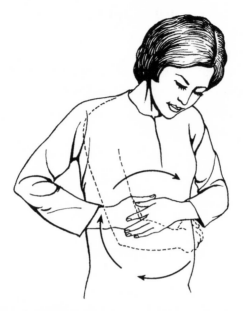

Abdominal Self-Massage

Abdominal self-massage can be performed daily for 10 to 20 minutes. Or it can be done anytime you feel discomfort. First warm your hands for a few minutes, by shaking them vigorously or by sitting on them. With your right hand, rub a small circle around your navel in a clockwise direction. Gradually increase the size of the circles. Experiment with different pressures. Now do the exercise with your left hand. Finally, perform the exercise with your left hand on top of your right hand.

Tip: This is a very effective exercise, but it must be practiced daily for its benefits to be felt, usually within thirty to sixty days.

to ten days after starting on the antibiotic, but they can develop after the drug has been stopped. The most serious form of antibiotic-associated diarrhea is pseudomembranous colitis, caused by overgrowth of the *Clostridium difficile* organism. Therefore, if you develop diarrhea from antibiotics, you should consult the physician who prescribed the drug. It may be necessary to switch to another medication.

Self Help

- Acidophilus/bifidus/FOS can be used to replenish healthy bacteria in the digestive tract (use dosage on the label)
- Digestive Harmony formula may be used as needed (2 to 3 tablets, 4 to 6 times per day) to improve absorption
- Eat baby food—it's easy to absorb
- Eat rice congee—1 cup of rice cooked in 6 to 8 cups water until a porridge results
- Use rehydration formulas or sports electrolyte drinks to replenish lost fluids

Professional Treatment

- In terms of Chinese medicine, antibiotics severely weaken the digestive system (stomach/spleen), therefore the formula Six Gentlemen (2 to 3 tablets TID) can be used to tonify the digestive system (by treating loose stools and fatigue) and to drain dampness
- Quiet Digestion (2 tablets TID or with each meal) helps treat food stagnation and improve absorption. With acute symptoms 3 tablets every hour may be administered
- Power Mushrooms (1 to 2 tablets TID) helps strengthen immunity
- Source Qi (3 to 5 tablets TID) addresses fatigue, chronic diarrhea, and cold signs
- Colostrum (1 to 3 tablets TID) can be used for acute or chronic diarrhea (hot or cold signs)
- Ease 2 (2 to 4 tablets TID) treats loose stools with irritability (liver Qi stagnation)

143

Case Studies

Case #1

Ken, a 64-year-old Japanese-American, reported a lifetime of diarrhea and tiredness after eating; particularly following lunch. Because of his age, he was referred to a gastroenterologist for tests; they were all normal. Ken was a tennis player and avid gardener. His diet consisted of mostly Japanese food. He seemed to have a sensitivity to fruits, which gave him gas. Traditional Chinese diagnosis found that his pulse was wiry and tongue red. He wanted to try herbs, which had previously helped him when he had kidney stones. He was advised to go on a soy-free and low fermented-food diet, eliminating soy, alcohol, dairy, fruits and high-fat foods for two weeks.

He was started on the herbal remedy Phellostatin, 1 tablet TID for the first week and then 2 tablets TID the second week. He was also given Colostroplex (2 tablets BID). Within two weeks his condition was alleviated. He was then to start reintroducing the foods he had previously eliminated. In subsequent weeks, he found that soy, milk, and alcohol contributed most to his diarrhea. After six weeks, Source Qi (3 tablets TID) was substituted for Phellostatin in order to address spleen Qi deficiency. Forty years of diarrhea would have damaged the digestive system and would be a major contributor to his fatigue. Colostroplex was reduced (1 tablet BID), Source Qi was started (3 tablets TID). He continued taking the Source Qi for three months and reported his afternoon fatigue greatly improved.

Case #2

Bob, 40, complained of chronic diarrhea and constant dull headache. His other symptoms included fatigue, low back pain, neck stiffness, night sweats, thirst, heartburn, and difficulty breathing. Before starting the herbal treatment, he was referred to a gastroenterologist for a complete work-up; however the tests turned out to be normal. Traditional Chinese diagnosis showed that his pulse was weak, and tongue pale. Hoping to relieve the headaches and neck stiffness, his acupuncturist consulted me and suggested a dispersing and heat clearing formula. It was obvious to me that the patient's headache was due to weakness from chronic diarrhea. My therapeutic strategy was to stop the diarrhea and tonify the body. Therefore, Source Qi was administered, 3 tablets TID the first week, 5 tablets TID thereafter. Later, when Bob was stronger, formulas such as Astra Essence could be used to tonify both the yin and the yang and to secure the essence. Rather than use herbs for the neck stiffness, I referred him for Tui Na (Chinese massage therapy). He was also counseled to take rice porridge (congee) with ginger once per day. After three weeks he experienced a 50 percent reduction in the number of trips to the bathroom. He also reported less fatigue. At this point, I recommended adding Ease 2 formula, which helps treat shoulder and neck tension, and rids the body of phlegm. In sum, Bob was taking Source Qi (3 tablets TID) with Ease 2 (3 tablets TID). After one month on the herbs, and undergoing weekly acupuncture and occasional massage therapy, all his symptoms improved.

Case #3:   Food Intolerance

Claire, a healthy looking 26-year-old, worked as a secretary. Hives were her primary reason for consultation. She also reported that foods such as pizza, chocolate, and fruit would "run right through," resulting in diarrhea and/or hives 15 minutes after eating, indicating that she had food intolerance. Other symptoms included constipation, feeling feverish (especially in the afternoon), and constant thirst. She had recently recovered from pneumonia, and indicated that as a child she had been sickly. Traditional Chinese diagnosis revealed that her pulse was thin, sinking, and fast. Her tongue was dry with red dots, and had a light gray

Electrolytes

Diarrhea causes dehydration, which depletes the body's stores of potassium. Dehydration and electrolyte imbalance (sodium and potassium ratio) manifest as fatigue. In the more severe form, you may get dizzy or have a headachy type of fatigue. Beverages such as Gatorade® or Recharge®, which are sold to athletes as electrolyte replacement drinks, are often useful in a pinch for severe diarrhea. Squash, apricots, oranges, and lima beans are high in potassium. Bananas are also rich in potassium, but they can have a moistening effect on the intestines, and should therefore be eaten in very small amounts during bouts of diarrhea. One of the most effective therapies for diarrhea as well as the common cold is homemade chicken soup, which is rich in potassium and low in sodium. However, it should be noted that packaged chicken soups are not effective because they contain too much sodium and not enough potassium. My personal observation and that of clients is that during flare-ups, a diet of homemade chicken soup and crackers is just about the best treatment. Tea, such as black or peppermint, is also helpful.

World Health Organization Electrolyte Replacement Formula: 3.5 g sodium chloride (salt), 2.5 g sodium bicarbonate (baking soda), 1.5 g potassium chloride, 20 g glucose, one liter (approximately 32 ounces) water.

Herbal Electrolyte Formula: 2 tbs peppermint, ½ tsp salt, ¼ tsp baking soda, ¼ tsp potassium chloride, 2 tbs molasses (brown sugar may be substituted in a pinch), 32 oz water. Steep the peppermint in 32 oz hot water for 15 to 20 minutes. Add the remaining items and stir until dissolved.

coating. I recommended Nine Flavor Tea (3 tablets TID), Coptis Purge Fire (1 tablet TID), and Colostroplex (1 to 2 tablets per day). I suggested that she give up cereal and soda for two weeks, to which she replied, "Now that you mention it, I actually do better when I don't eat cereal in the morning" (most cereal grains have allergens). One week later, she reported no diarrhea, and fewer outbreaks of hives. She still had thirst and some facial flushing. She continued on the same herbal protocol. Three weeks later, I recommended increasing the dosage of Coptis Purge Fire (3 tablets TID), while maintaining the same dosage of Nine Flavor Tea. She had also started drinking more water, eating healthier, and at the next visit reported no more diarrhea or hives.

Diverticulosis/Diverticulitis

Half the U.S. population over age 60 has diverticulosis, a condition in which diverticula—small pouches of intestinal lining—protrude inward from the large intestine. It is thought that diverticula form as a result of spasm of the muscles in the intestinal wall. The spasms cause the lining of the intestines to bulge through the weakest area of the muscle, much as a weak, bulging spot might develop in a defective tire or basketball. Diverticula may be caused by lack of fiber in the diet; their occurrence is very rare in the developing countries, where grains, fruits, and vegetables are the main foods consumed. The theory is that adding bulk to the stool gives the muscles a mass to work against, decreasing the likelihood of spasm, in the same way that well-toned skeletal muscles are less likely to cramp, than ones that are not exercised regularly.

The symptoms of diverticulosis may include lower abdominal pain and cramps, gas, bloating, irregular bowel movements, and bleeding from the rectum. Diverticula are usually discovered after symptoms appear, or they may be detected by X-rays, or during endoscopy for other complaints. The symptoms of diverticulitis, an inflammation of the diverticula, may include fever, pain, and abdominal tenderness, usually in the lower left part of the abdomen.

Conventional medical treatment for diverticulosis is to consume more fiber, and to take psyllium supplements. Diverticulitis can have serious medical complications, and patients with diverticulosis who develop lower abdominal pain with spasm or fever should consult a physician. Routine cases are treated with bed rest, a liquid diet, and antibiotics. The symptoms of colon cancer and appendicitis are similar to those of diverticulosis or diverticulitis, and anyone with acute abdominal pain should seek out a physician for a definitive diagnosis.

Professional Treatment

- Six Gentlemen (3 tablets TID) can be used to prevent diverticulosis if a patient has fatigue and cold signs
- Isatis Cooling (3 to 5 tablets TID) can be administered for pain as this formula has anti-inflammatory properties
- Aquilaria 22 (1 to 3 tablets TID) can be used to promote circulation to the intestine and to treat constipation
- Formula H (3 to 5 tablets TID) can help treat rectal bleeding (if you do have rectal bleeding be sure to see your medical doctor for an exam)

Case Study

Eleanor, 60, had abdominal cramping and constipation due to diverticulitis. Traditional Chinese diagnosis found her pulse to be thin, wiry, and tongue pale with a red border, suggesting heat in the liver. She also said she felt hot in the afternoon although the weather was usually cold. I recommended a combination of Isatis

Cooling (2 tablets QID) and Aquilaria 22 (2 tablets QID). In addition, I advised her to drink chamomile tea, 3 cups per day. After two weeks Eleanor noticed less abdominal pain. Since the hot signs had also abated, I recommended she finish the bottle of Isatis Cooling and continue taking Aquilaria 22, which she did faithfully for several months. Then as the weather began changing and she was showing signs of a cold condition, the formula Six Gentlemen (2 tablets TID) was added. Eleanor has been very satisfied with the herbal therapy, as her abdominal pain has been alleviated and her bowel movements have become more normal.

Fecal Incontinence

Fecal incontinence is the inability to control bowel movements. This condition is common in seniors, when the muscles and ligaments that control defecation become less efficient. Incontinence can also result from an abscess or inflammation in the rectum, anus, or perianal area, or from trauma, injury, or surgery; as well as a nervous disorder, such as diabetic gastroparesis. Chronic diarrhea may be a contributing factor. A bowel-training program may be started, which involves sitting on the toilet for a certain time every day. Increasing dietary fiber helps to produce a more normal stool. Biofeedback, self-hypnosis, and surgery may also be helpful.

Professional Treatment

- Formulas such as Colostroplex (1 to 3 tablets TID) and Source Qi (3 to 5 tablets TID) help reduce the frequency of bowel movements
- Source Qi aids in building up muscle tone in the rectal area, as several of the formula's herbs are traditionally used to strengthen the muscles

Case Studies

Case #1

A colleague passed this case on to me.

Due to her fear of incontinence, Joann was housebound for over two years. Her condition was unresponsive to conventional and alternative methods. One day, there was an electrical fire in her house, which necessitated her going over to the neighbor's in order to contact the fire department. She waited outside for over two hours while the firemen put out the fire. It wasn't until five o'clock on this hectic day that she had her first bowel movement, not even realizing that she hadn't thought about having diarrhea all day. From that point on her condition turned around.

This case demonstrates how if the mind is otherwise occupied, the body will be free of symptoms. This is why having a mission in life is so important (see Chapter Two).

Case #2

Eva, 78, first experienced incontinence after chemotherapy treatments for stomach cancer. She also confided that she was very worried about her adult son, who was a drug addict. Traditional Chinese diagnosis found that her pulse was sinking and thin, and her tongue was pale, flabby, and red at the tip. We recommended Source Qi formula (5 tablets TID). However, because it was difficult for her to swallow 5 tablets, 3 times a day, her daughter made a tea out of the tablets. After four weeks, Alma noticed that she was no longer experiencing spontaneous evacuations, which greatly improved her self esteem. Since she was a spiritual woman, we also encouraged her to pray, in order to alleviate some of the emotional stress associated with her son.

Gallstones and Gallbladder Inflammation

The gallbladder stores bile, which is manufactured in the liver, until it is needed in the small intestine to aid in the digestion of fats. Under some conditions, stones form in the gallbladder. The stones are usually composed of cholesterol, a normal constituent of bile. When they block the flow of bile, pain in the upper or mid-right abdomen results. This pain is usually worse after a fatty meal, when bile flow through the gallbladder ducts is stimulated. Other symptoms such as bloating, gas, and belching may occur. If gallstones run in your family there is a higher chance that you will develop them. Being female, overweight, and over 40 years old also increases the likelihood of developing gallstones.

Common surgical treatments for gallstones include removal of the gallbladder, removal of the stones themselves, or widening of the sphincter between the gall ducts and intestine, in order to allow easier passage of the stones. Drugs, or other techniques to dissolve or break up the stones, can also be used. Blockage of the bile duct, or infection of the gallbladder (cholecystitis) that does not respond to antibiotics, may require emergency removal of the gallbladder.

Serious gallbladder problems are usually preceded by years of symptoms of indigestion. Treatment of these symptoms by natural methods, including proper diet and exercise habits, can prevent more serious developments.

Professional Treatment

- GB-6 formula (3 tablets QID) is used to treat gallstones and to prevent their formation in those who eat excessive amounts of fats; it is also used to treat gallbladder inflammation
- The adjunct formula Ecliptex (2 tablets QID) is used to address liver Qi stagnation, and liver toxicity

- For overweight patients, consider Astra Diet Tea (1 cup following each meal) and Astra 18 Diet Fuel (3 tablets ½ hour before meals with two large glasses of water)

Case Studies

Case #1

An overweight male in his early 50s came to our clinic complaining of radiating pain that worsened after eating foods with a high fat content. Ultrasound diagnosis showed that he had several gallstones, averaging 7 to 8 millimeters each. His pulse was wiry and tongue red with a yellow coating. A combination of GB-6 (3 tablets QID) and Ecliptex (2 tablets QID) was recommended. He was counseled to cut down on dietary fats and to start an exercise program. After two months his pain had decreased significantly and he had lost about 5 pounds. I told him to eat a carrot any time he was hungry, instead of his usual crackers and pastries. Within six months his ultrasound examination revealed no gallstones.

Case #2

An overweight woman in her early 40s was diagnosed by ultrasound to have eight gallstones, averaging 4 millimeters each. She complained of radiating pain in the upper abdomen. Her pulse was thin and slightly wiry, and her tongue had a yellow coating. She was put on GB-6, Ecliptex, and Astra 18 (2 tablets TID of each formula). Within four months all the stones were reduced in size by 50 percent.

Case #3

A male patient in his early 40s, who was approximately 30 pounds overweight and had a fondness for overeating, had recently gone to the hospital emergency room for abdominal pain following the consumption of a heavy banquet meal. He was advised to cut down his fat intake and was then sent home. His main symptoms were epigastric discomfort after breakfast (the discomfort sometimes lasted the entire day), and nausea, which was eliminated by eating. Traditional Chinese diagnosis showed he had a weak pulse, and greasy tongue coating. I suggested Astra Diet Tea (1 cup after each meal), which soothes the digestive system and GB-6 (3 tablets TID). The first day after taking the herbs he noticed that the nausea and discomfort were eliminated.

Case #4
Gloria, 76, complained of phantom pain in her gallbladder, radiating to the shoulder, despite having had her gallbladder removed over ten years earlier. She also suffered fatigue. Traditional Chinese diagnosis revealed that her pulse was sinking, though slightly wiry, and her tongue had a thick, sticky coating. She was advised to take GB-6 (3 tablets TID), which totally relieved her pain after one week. Thereafter, she continued using GB-6 as needed.

Gastritis

Gastritis is an inflammation of the stomach lining. The main symptom is upper abdominal discomfort. Nausea, vomiting, and diarrhea may also be evident. In otherwise asymptomatic cases, gastric bleeding may be present and is characterized by blood in the vomit, or by black, tarry stools; this is a serious symptom usually requiring hospitalization.

There are various causes of gastritis. Medications, particularly those for pain, can lead to gastritis. This condition can also result from inflammation due to burns or trauma, and from poor circulation due to surgery or shock. Or, it may be caused by the *Helicobacter pylori* bacteria, which many in the medical community now regard as the main cause of gastritis and ulcers, and treat accordingly with a combination of antacids and antibiotics. Contributing factors of gastritis include cigarette smoking and alcohol. Also, gastritis can be associated with vitamin B_{12} deficiency, which is common in senior citizens. Diagnosis of gastritis is based on presenting symptoms and tests as deemed necessary by your health professional.

Self Help

- Use slippery elm (1 to 3 teaspoons) along with oatmeal in the morning and later with a glass of hot or lukewarm water, once or twice per day
- Supplement with vitamin B_{12} if deficient; use sublingual B_{12} (1,000 to 2,000 mcg per day), or obtain injections from your doctor (injections may be necessary when hydrochloric acid secretion in the stomach is insufficient)

Professional Treatment

- Isatis Cooling (3 to 5 tablets TID) can be used to soothe inflammation and speed up the healing process
- Quiet Digestion (2 tablets TID or as needed) helps restore the acid/alkaline balance in the stomach
- Clearing (3 tablets TID) helps reduce stomach inflammation and generate fluids

Gastrointestinal Bleeding

Gastrointestinal bleeding is marked by dark, black, or red blood in the stool, or by vomiting of blood. The most common causes are peptic ulcer, gastritis, bleeding in the esophagus, tears in the esophagus or upper stomach, as well as tumors, polyps, and diverticula in the colon, or hemorrhoids. All cases of gastrointestinal bleeding require a prompt diagnosis, and if bleeding is excessive, emergency medical care is warranted.

Professional Treatment

- Formula H (5 tablets TID) may be used to relieve bloody stools
- Quiet Digestion and Ease Plus (2 to 3 tablets of each formula QID) help alleviate vomiting of blood; for obvious fever or other heat signs, use Ease Plus and Coptis Purge Fire (2 to 3 tablets of each formula QID)

Heartburn

(See Indigestion and Reflux Esophagitis)

Hemorrhoids

Hemorrhoids are very common. Both diarrhea and constipation can cause and aggravate the problem. Hemorrhoids are varicose veins in the rectum. They can lead to rectal pain, bleeding, and itching, or they can be relatively symptomless. Sometimes hemorrhoids can prevent the anus from closing fully, causing soiling of the underwear. Fissures, cracks in the skin around the anus can also form. External hemorrhoids are found outside the anus, often with accompanying pain. Internal hemorrhoids occur inside the rectum and do not cause pain, unless they are prolapsed. Prolapsing can close off the anus, and can be extremely painful. Bleeding from the rectum can also signal rectal cancer or polyps, so medical diagnosis is a must if you have this symptom. Surgery is necessary if a blood clot develops in a hemorrhoid.

Treat hemorrhoids by increasing dietary fiber, avoiding straining during bowel movements, and by taking warm Sitz baths.

Self Help

- Sitz bath: Fill the bathtub with 4 inches of warm water. Add ¼ cup of Epsom salts. Sit in this mixture for 10 minutes, 3 or 4 times per day for best results
- Add a tea made of comfrey or yarrow to the Sitz bath by first steeping 4 ounces (112 g) of the dry herbs in 32 ounces (1 liter) of boiling water for 10 minutes. Strain and add to the bath
- Try stoneroot (collinsonia), 3 to 6 grams per day internally, and use topical remedies found at your pharmacy containing witch hazel, followed by application of vitamin E topically

Professional Treatment

Formula H (3 tablets TID) is an effective herbal remedy, as it contains anti-inflammatory (heat clearing) and pain relieving properties

Case Study

Renee, a 32-year-old businesswoman, complained of internal hemorrhoids causing burning, itching, and straining upon bowel movements. She also experienced PMS and occasional vaginal yeast infections, and had a history of asthma. Traditional Chinese diagnosis revealed that her pulse was superficial and wiry, and her tongue had red spots, was pale in the center, and had a thin white coating. I advised her to use over-the-counter remedies for hemorrhoids daily, including ointment and witch hazel pads. The following herbal formulas were suggested: Woman's Balance (2 tablets QID) and Formula H (2 tablets QID). The hemorrhoids and accompanying symptoms were quickly brought under control. I had her follow up with the formulas Calm Spirit (2 tablets QID) and Woman's Balance (2 tablets QID) to help treat the underlying condition, which was stress and anxiety. I also recommended a meditation break during her twelve-hour workday.

Hepatitis

Hepatitis is an inflammation of the liver. It is commonly caused by viral infection, drugs, alcohol, and toxic agents. Acute viral hepatitis is characterized by jaundice (yellowing of the skin and eyes), fever, fatigue, tenderness in the upper right abdomen, nausea and vomiting, dark urine, and pale stools. The specific viruses that cause viral hepatitis include hepatitis A, B, C, D, and E viruses. Hepatitis A and E are highly contagious and are spread by contact with fecal matter, via contaminated fingers, water, or food. Raw shellfish tainted with the virus can also cause Hepatitis A. Hepatitis A is found the world over, while hepatitis E has been responsible for outbreaks in Mexico, Afghanistan, Algeria, India, and Burma. Hepatitis B, C, and D are transmitted by contaminated blood on infected needles, through blood transfusion, or during sexual intercourse. Hepatitis B may be transmitted to an infant at childbirth if the mother is infected. It is postulated that Hepatitis C may also be spread through shared razors, body piercing, tattooing, and by straws used during cocaine snorting. Conventional medical treatment involves rest and a nourishing diet, since there is no specific treatment for acute hepatitis. When a cause is known, such as a medication or toxic substance, then stopping the exposure is key in avoiding further liver damage.

Chronic hepatitis results when an individual fails to recover fully from acute hepatitis, and the liver cell damage and inflammation continue. In some cases there are no symptoms at all, in others a slight feeling of being ill, while yet others have recurrent acute episodes. There are different types of chronic hepatitis. One kind is due to heavy alcohol consumption, and in other types the cause is an autoimmune disorder, a reaction to a medication, or a metabolic condition affecting the liver. In terms of treatment, conventional medicine recommends abstinence from alcohol, and for autoimmune causes the use of corticosteroids, immune suppressive drugs, recombinant human interferon alfa-2b, and liver transplant if the liver has been severely damaged. Prolonged bedrest has not been shown to be beneficial, meaning that some activity should be maintained, albeit modified according to the patient's symptoms.

Hepatitis is a disease that can be prevented through vaccines and good hygiene habits. Vaccines are available for hepatitis A and B, and are recommended for travelers to areas where hepatitis is rampant such as much of Asia, Africa, and Eastern Europe. Type B vaccine is particularly recommended for health care workers, persons with multiple sexual partners, dialysis patients, and children born to infected mothers. Practicing good hygiene is the simplest and most effective way to prevent contracting diseases such as hepatitis. Thorough hand washing must be undertaken after going to the bathroom (following both urination and bowel movements), after changing diapers, and before and after handling food. When traveling outside the U.S. and western Europe, drink only boiled, bottled, or filtered water, eat only cooked foods, and peel all fruit. Injections should be done only with sterile or disposable needles. Ask about sterilization if you are getting your body pierced or tattooed. Request disposable acupuncture needles.

Self Help

- For the treatment of viral and chronic hepatitis, Ralph Golan, MD, recommends powdered buffered vitamin C to bowel tolerance.[3] Take 10 g the first day; if you get loose stools reduce the dosage by ⅓, if no loose stools increase the dosage by 5 g per day until you have loose stools, then reduce to the highest dosage that does not cause loose stools. A maintenance dose of 1 to 5 g per day may be considered for long-term use. A broad spectrum antioxidant is also helpful (for dosages see Chapter Three)
- Alpha Lipoic acid (100 to 200 mg TID) is recommended by holistic doctors
- Milk thistle extract (100 to 200 mg TID) can be taken to improve liver function

Professional Treatment

- Coptis Purge Fire (3 tablets 4 to 6 times per day) can be used to treat acute viral hepatitis accompanied by fever, jaundice, and dark urine. Reduce dosage if loose stools occur. For high fever add Clear Heat formula (3 tablets 4 to 6 times per day)
- A combination of Ecliptex (2 to 3 tablets TID) and Clear Heat (1 tablet TID if no heat signs, 3 tablets TID with heat signs) is useful long term for chronic hepatitis. Ecliptex helps reduce liver enzymes; Clear Heat is beneficial as it is comprised of antiviral herbs
- For abdominal swelling and edema use Drain Dampness (2 to 3 tablets TID); this formula should be used cautiously for patients on pharmaceutical diuretics, as it contains natural diuretics
- With fatigue used Ecliptex (2 to 3 tablets TID) and Astra Isatis (3 tablets TID)

- For anemia and tiredness consider Ecliptex (2 to 3 tablets TID) and Marrow Plus (3 tablets TID)
- Some holistic doctors recommend thymus preparations as part of an overall regimen for chronic hepatitis (use as directed)

Case Studies

Case #1

Melinda, a 64-year-old part-time cook, came in with a diagnosis of chronic hepatitis C, cirrhosis, and inoperable liver cancer. In addition, she was about 80 pounds overweight, with massive edema of the legs and stomach. She was very fatigued and had muscle and joint pain, however she was able to continue working part-time. Traditional Chinese diagnosis found that her pulse was thin and sinking, and her tongue was wet and red. Our first approach was to reduce the edema using the formulas Drain Dampness and Regeneration (starting dosage was 2 tablets TID of each formula, increased to 3 tablets TID of each formula by the third week). After one month, the swelling in her legs was significantly better. At this point, her pulse was weak in the kidney position, and her tongue remained wet and red. She continued with the herbs. Two weeks later she came to the clinic in an exhausted state. It turned out she had volunteered to work an extra shift. There was still some edema, although not as severe as when she first came in. However, her abdomen was very bloated. Her pulse was weak, and tongue red and no longer wet. The day previously she had seen her medical doctor, who diagnosed her with ascites. Therefore, with this visit her regimen was altered: Regeneration was stopped, and Aquilaria 22 (2 tablets TID) was added, while Drain Dampness was maintained (same dosage). After six weeks on the new protocol her abdomen was less bloated and the edema had dissipated some. Her pulse was weak and slippery, and her tongue red and dry (i.e., no longer wet). She was then advised to resume the original herbal protocol of Drain Dampness and Regeneration (3 tablets of each TID). Today, she continues utilizing herbs and conventional medical care. She has more energy, reduced fat, and less edema and bloating than when she first came to the clinic.

Case #2

Maria, a 40-year-old housecleaner, had been diagnosed with chronic hepatitis C. She also had anemia and complained of exhaustion. She had refused interferon treatment because of the side effects and the low success rate. She was unable to take the iron preparation recommended by her doctor, as it was constipating. Traditional Chinese diagnosis revealed that her pulse was slightly wiry and weak in the kidney position, and her tongue was reddish purple with a geographic coating. I recommended the formulas Ecliptex and Marrow Plus (2 tablets TID of each formula the first two weeks, then 3 tablets TID of each thereafter). Ecliptex regenerates the liver and has been found to reduce liver enzymes in many patients. Marrow Plus replenishes the blood and Qi and is currently being studied in an anemia clinical trial. Maria was also advised to switch to a liquid iron preparation, to avoid constipation from iron supplementation. After two months on the herbal formulas, she reported having significantly more energy. She remains on the herbs.

Herpes Simplex of the Esophagus

The herpes simplex virus can cause inflammation and ulcers in the esophagus, leading to such symptoms as acid regurgitation and heartburn. Acyclovir is the conventional drug treatment.

Professional Treatments

- The antiviral formula Clear Heat (3 to 4 tablets, up to 6 times per day) is effective
- Astra Isatis formula (3 tablets QID) is effective in preventing and reducing the frequency of herpes outbreaks. Combine Astra Isatis with Power Mushrooms (1 to 2 tablets QID) when cold signs are present; for heat signs combine with Clear Heat (1 to 2 tablets QID)

Hiatal Hernia

This is a condition in which a part of the stomach protrudes upward into the chest through an opening in the diaphragm. It tends to occur in obese people, especially upper middle-aged people, and in smokers. Most patients are asymptomatic, but in some, spasms of the esophagus can result in acid reflux and bloating after meals. A special chiropractic adjustment technique can help relieve hiatal hernia.

Professional Treatment

- Quiet Digestion (2 tablets TID or QID) contains enzymes to help move food through the digestive system and eliminate bloating. It is often combined with Ease Plus (2 tablets QID)
- Clear Phlegm *(Wen Dan Tang)* can be used if phlegm signs are present (1 to 3 tablets TID)
- Use SPZM (2 tablets QID) with Ease Plus (2 tablets QID) for abdominal spasms
- For spasms accompanied by loose stools use SPZM (2 tablets QID) and Ease 2 (2 tablets QID)

Hiccups

Hiccups are involuntary contractions of the diaphragm. They are most likely to occur after eating a heavy meal or from eating and/or drinking too fast. Hiccups can also be caused by stress. In rare instances the condition can arise due to irritation of the diaphragm or of the phrenic nerves that supply it. In most cases the attacks are self resolving. However, there are extremely rare cases when prolonged bouts of hiccups can lead to exhaustion, and may require medication or even surgery.

Self Help

- Massage the back of mouth with a cotton swab by moving it back and forth for about 1 minute
- Suck on a sugar cube
- Swallow three tablespoons of vinegar
- When accompanied by cold signs, use clove tea by first boiling ¼ to 1 teaspoon of cloves for 15 minutes, consume while hot
- For long-standing recurrent hiccups, take biotin, a B vitamin

Professional Treatment

- In Chinese medicine hiccups are considered "rebellious Qi," for which the formula Ease Plus (2 to 3 tablets TID) is effective
- Cir-Q (1 to 2 tablets QID) contains cloves and other herbs used to move stagnant Qi, and can be administered as an adjunct to Ease Plus
- For accompanying heat signs use Ease Plus and Coptis Purge Fire (2 tablets of each formula TID to QID)
- For accompanying indigestion use Ease Plus along with Quiet Digestion (2 tablets of each formula QID)

- Acupuncture is often effective in treating hiccups (see Appendix C)

Case Studies

Case #1

Neil, 43, had been having recurrent bouts of hiccups for two weeks. Traditional Chinese diagnosis revealed that his pulse was sinking and wiry, and tongue flabby with a dirty yellow coating. I recommended that he obtain a medical evaluation to rule out any pathological causes. He was advised to drink clove tea (3 cups per day), to take Ease Plus (3 tablets TID), and to apply the cotton swab technique. The hiccups were resolved after a few days.

Case #2

Ron, a 42-year-old plumber, complained of frequent episodes of hiccups for the previous two years. He had seen numerous health professionals but without relief. Traditional Chinese diagnosis found that his pulse was wiry and rapid, his tongue red with a gray coating. He was administered Ease Plus, Coptis Purge Fire, and Clear Heat (2 tablets QID of each formula), and instructed to apply the cotton swab technique. Within the first day of taking the herbs, he experienced less frequency in the hiccups, and after one week they were eliminated.

HIV-Related Digestive Disorders

HIV patients are likely to have many digestive symptoms as a result of opportunistic parasitic, viral, or bacterial infections, or from the side effects of medications that they take. An experienced herbalist can administer the following protocols. While undertaking these herbal treatments, patients should also be monitored by physicians experienced in the treatment of HIV.

Professional Treatment

- For occasional digestive symptoms, Quiet Digestion (2 tablets TID or as needed) is effective in reducing the side effects of some medications
- For cryptosporidiosis, administer Source Qi (3 to 5 tablets TID) and Artestatin (start at 1 tablet per day and increase by 1 tablet daily until a maximum of 6 to 9 tablets are taken)
- For cytomegalovirus intestinal infection, administer Colostroplex (2 to 6 tablets daily) and Clear Heat (2 to 4 tablets QID)
- Parasitic infections such as giardiasis and toxoplasmosis are treated using formulas such as Artestatin (start at 1 tablet daily and increase by 1 tablet to 1 to 3 tablets TID), along with Aquilaria 22 (2 to 3 tablets TID)
- For chronic diarrhea unaffected by *Cryptosporidia,* and an absence of fever and rectal bleeding, Source Qi alone can be administered. For fever and rectal bleeding, consider Formula H (3 to 5 tablets TID), along with Colostroplex (1 to 3 tablets TID)
- For weight loss, a combination of Source Qi (3 to 5 tablets TID) and Colostroplex (1 to 3 tablets TID) are recommended. Colostroplex improves absorption and assimilation of nutrients, which in addition to a high protein diet can promote weight gain
- For pancreatitis with fever, jaundice-type symptoms, bitter taste in the mouth, and nausea, use Coptis Purge Fire (3 tablets 4 to 6 times a day); with boring pain add Channel Flow (2 tablets QID); with heat signs add Clear Heat (2 to 3 tablets 4 to 6 times a day)
- For hepatitis, consider Ecliptex (2 tablets TID) and Clear Heat (1 to 3 tablets TID; if heat signs are present, use a higher dosage of 3 tablets TID)
- Long-term administration of Enhance (5 tablets QID) or

165

Astra Isatis (3 tablets QID) can be used to address fatigue and to improve quality of life. A double-blind study at the University of California, San Francisco, found that Enhance helped improve quality of life of HIV patients

Case Studies

Case #1

Rafael, a man in his early 40s, had cryptosporidiosis and AIDS, and was given less than one year to live by his doctor. He had eighteen to twenty-five watery bowel movements a day. His other symptoms were depression, nausea, fatigue, lack of appetite, and dizziness when standing. Traditional Chinese diagnosis found that his pulse was weak, and tongue pale and wet. He started on 3 tablets TID of Source Qi and 1 tablet per day of Artestatin. As his intestinal gas increased after starting on the herbs, he was advised to add Quiet Digestion, 1 to 2 tablets TID. His dosages of Source Qi and Artestatin were gradually increased to 5 tablets TID and 1 tablet TID, respectively. He also continued with the 2 tablets TID of Quiet Digestion. As a result of this regimen, he was having less than five loosely formed stools per day. His general outlook improved considerably over the next three months, at the end of which he was having only three bowel movements per day. He also reported that smoking marijuana before eating improved his appetite.

Case #2

Following a trip to Mexico, Elliot, a man in his late 30s with HIV, was diagnosed with chronic shigellosis. The main symptoms were abdominal pain and liquid stools with mucus. The antibiotic he was prescribed increased the diarrhea and abdominal cramping. He was then put on a different antibiotic. When he consulted me, he was severely fatigued and having over ten liquid stools per day. Traditional Chinese diagnosis revealed that his pulse was weak, and tongue pale. I recommended a combination of Source Qi (5 tablets TID) and Quiet Digestion (2 tablets every 3 hours for the first 3 days, and 2 tablets QID or more if needed, thereafter). I also recommended taking PB 8 acidophilus bifidus (4 capsules) at bedtime. Five weeks later, his stools and energy were back to normal.

Intestinal Gas (Flatulence)

It is natural to have gas in the colon. It is usually expelled during a bowel movement. However, some people have an excessive amount of gas, and are bothered by it throughout the day. Intestinal gas is primarily composed of oxygen, nitrogen, hydrogen, carbon dioxide, and methane. Oxygen and nitrogen are found in the air we breathe, whereas the other gases are primarily the result of bacterial fermentation in the large intestine. Some foods that may cause excessive gas are beans, peas, wheat, oats, bran, brussels sprouts, cabbage, corn, rutabaga, and dairy products. From a naturopathic point of view, excessive gas may be an indication of *Candida* overgrowth. Candidiasis can be worsened by eating excessive amounts of fermented and yeast-containing foods, such as soy sauce, beer, bread, sugar, fruit juice, or fruit.

Intestinal gas can be aggravated when dietary fiber intake is increased, and sometimes it occurs when taking herbal remedies one is unaccustomed to. Eating too fast and chewing gum can contribute to gas as well, because of swallowed air. Therefore, eat food slowly and chew thoroughly. Carbonated beverages and sugar substitutes can also contribute. In terms of Chinese medicine, gas is usually due to diet, stress, and spleen Qi deficiency that is accompanied by dampness. Over-the-counter remedies should not be taken to relieve or prevent gas, because there is no strong evidence that they are effective.

Self Help

* Peppermint tea may be taken several times per day
* Use the formula Digestive Harmony (2 tablets as needed) to help expel or reduce gas
* Activated charcoal may be taken short term. Follow instructions carefully. Do not take at the same time as other medications

Professional Treatment

* Anti-*Candida* diets are often very effective. In addition, anti-*Candida* herbal formulas such as Phellostatin (1 to 2 tablets TID) are helpful, particularly when combined with symptomatic formulas such as Quiet Digestion. Quiet Digestion (2 tablets every 4 hours) may be used alone for gas pain
* As mentioned above, Chinese medicine considers excessive gas due to weak spleen function, thus formulas such as Six Gentlemen (3 tablets TID) may be combined with Quiet Digestion (2 tablets TID), particularly if the patient has a weak pulse and complains of fatigue
* For cold signs, consider Stomach Tabs alone (3 tablets TID), or with Six Gentlemen (3 tablets TID)
* With stress use Heavenly Water, Woman's Balance, or Ease 2 (3 tablets TID for each formula); for PMS use Woman's Balance or Heavenly Water (same dosages)

Case Studies

Case #1
A female patient in her mid–30s complained of frequent intestinal gas, nausea, severe PMS, fatigue, and low back pain. She usually had a glass or two of wine each night, and had a fondness

for sweets. Traditional Chinese diagnosis revealed that her pulse was wiry, and tongue swollen, wet, and red around the edges. Before recommending any herbal formulas, I suggested she give up alcohol—or have it only occasionally—and instead, practice meditation after work. I also recommended cutting out sweets, as this would reduce both the PMS and intestinal gas. She was then given Woman's Balance and Quiet Digestion (2 tablets TID of each formula), as well as Adrenosen, to be taken symptomatically for fatigue. After two months she reported more energy, less gas, and that the PMS was less severe. She still had lingering back pain. At this point, she discontinued Quiet Digestion, was given Astra Essence (2 tablets TID) to tonify the body, and continued on Woman's Balance.

Case #2

A male sales representative, 35, came to our clinic complaining of chronic gas, abdominal bloating, and fatigue. He had already tried digestive enzymes and acidophilus. Traditional Chinese diagnosis found that his pulse was weak, and tongue wet. He was put on a combination of Quiet Digestion and Six Gentlemen (2 tablets QID of each formula) and was counseled not to consume cold drinks or foods, and to decrease his intake of fatty and fried foods. Within two weeks the gas was significantly reduced.

Case #3

A male, 27, was diagnosed with irritable bowel syndrome. His main symptoms were bloating, loose stools, and excessive gas in the afternoon and evening. Traditional Chinese diagnosis revealed that his pulse was thin and wiry, and tongue had a thick gray coating. I suggested following the Digestive Clearing Diet (see Chapter Five). In addition, he was given Phellostatin (2 tablets before each meal) and Colostroplex (2 tablets BID between meals). Within one month, nearly all symptoms had been reduced by 90 percent.

Irritable Bowel Syndrome (IBS)

Irritable bowel syndrome (IBS) is also known as spastic colon, spastic colitis, mucous colitis, nervous stomach, nervous diarrhea, and functional bowel disease. It is estimated that up to 22 percent of the U.S. population has IBS, either occasionally or persistently. There are some estimates indicating that this condition is the second most common reason for absence from work or school. IBS is usually triggered by diet and emotionally stressful situations. Symptoms include bouts of diarrhea, diarrhea alternating with constipation, constipation, excessive gas, belching, and abdominal pain. It is experienced as "gas pain" by many sufferers. Considerable anxiety is associated with the constant urgent need to go to the bathroom. It can be humiliating to have to get up several times during dinner at a restaurant to go to the bathroom, or fear that one will not make it to the bathroom in time while engaged in a business meeting or other important activity. Despite this, IBS is actually one of the more treatable digestive conditions, and responds particularly well to exercise, stress reduction, and dietary modification. The conventional medical approach is to use fiber supplements in powder form, in addition to sedatives or relaxants. If your IBS began after drinking untreated water, or a trip to the third world, consider herbal treatment for parasites (see "Parasites," later in this chapter).

Self Help

- Drink peppermint or chamomile tea throughout the day, at least 3 large cups per day
- Drink relaxing tea blends that contain the above-mentioned herbs, along with passionflower and valerian
- Digestive Harmony formula (2 tablets TID), which reduces

gas and treats gas pain, may be used to help food assimilate more easily. It may also be taken with meals

Professional Treatment

- For IBS, Quiet Digestion (2 tablets TID, or as needed) can be taken before and after meals. It is used to help food assimilate more easily, especially when one feels food is "stuck" in the GI tract
- Isatis Cooling (3 to 5 tablets TID) is used for stabbing cramps and heat signs
- Woman's Balance (3 tablets TID) is used for stress and hormonal imbalance
- Use Ease Plus and Calm Spirit (2 tablets TID of each formula) for anxiety and accompanying constipation
- Use Ease 2 (3 tablets TID) for stress, shoulder and neck tension, and loose stools
- Use Colostroplex (1 to 2 tablets TID) for diarrhea; reduce dosage if constipation occurs

Case Studies

Case #1

An 11-year-old girl developed IBS following her parents' divorce. Her condition was so severe that she was unable to control her bowels, resulting in spontaneous episodes in public. Traditional Chinese diagnosis found that her pulse was wiry and rapid, and tongue red. She was put on Colostroplex (2 tablets BID) and referred for acupuncture to reduce stress symptoms. According to her practitioner, there was dramatic improvement within four weeks.

Case #2

A 44-year-old nurse with a lifelong history of "nervous stomach" became aware that her digestive symptoms were not confined to stressful events. She had urgent diarrhea in the morning, abdominal bloating one hour after eating meals, a bitter taste in her mouth, thirst without desire to drink, PMS, constant fatigue, and nighttime urination. Traditional Chinese diagnosis found that her tongue was thin and wiry, and tongue red on the edges and pale in the center. I suggested she embark on an exercise program. She was given Colostroplex (2 tablets BID) as well as Woman's Balance and Gastrodia Relieve Wind (2 tablets QID of each formula) during ovulation. In addition, she used Cramp Bark Plus (2 tablets QID) for painful menstruation, and Astra Essence and Six Gentlemen postmenstrually (2 tablets of each QID). After one month, she complained of constipation, so Colostroplex was reduced to 1 tablet BID. Since she admitted to not taking the recommended dosage of the other herbs, I stressed the importance of an adequate dosage in order to ensure the swiftest possible results. After the second month, she reported no PMS, less nighttime urination, and greater energy. She said she felt better than she had in years.

Case #3

Debbie, 35, works in sales and travels constantly. She has had diarrhea for a number of years and has undergone a battery of conventional medical tests. All results were negative, and her condition was given the medical diagnosis of IBS. Traditional Chinese diagnosis found that her pulse was wiry and rapid, and tongue red and dry. I suggested that she reduce her intake of greasy and fried foods, as well as begin a stress reduction and exercise program. Colostroplex (2 tablets BID) was recommended, and within two weeks her stools were solid. A week later, however, she reported that she was experiencing constipation. The dosage was then reduced to 1 tablet BID. At this time, she also began taking Woman's Balance (2 tablets TID) to regulate the body's energy and to reduce stress and PMS. She was doing well until she took an extended road trip for two weeks, during which she ran out of Colostroplex. When she returned home she resumed the Colostroplex at 2 tablets BID, but reported that the diarrhea had recurred.

When Debbie came in for another consultation, I asked whether she was following my dietary, stress reduction, and exercise suggestions. She reported that she had until she went on the business trip. I gave her some suggestions based on my own experience. I pointed out that she had to commit to the program, even when she was on the road. I recommended that whenever possible she stay in hotels with a swimming pool or gym, and if such facilities are not available usually the hotel can refer guests to a nearby health club. I also suggested that when on the road, she seek out a health food store with a deli, where she could have more control over what she ate, as opposed to eating rich restaurant food. Finally, in terms of her herbal regimen, Source Qi formula (3 tablets TID) was added to address her exhaustion. I indicated that she could regulate the herbs and supplements according to her symptoms. The Source Qi formula gave her more energy and quickly improved her diarrhea.

Case #4

Claire, a 48-year-old who had experienced IBS symptoms since she was fourteen, was diagnosed with candidiasis by a holistic medical doctor. Her history included sensitivity to dairy and wheat, and flare-ups of intense intestinal pain and watery bowels, which left her exhausted for a couple of days. Since she was exhibiting many heat signs, including bleeding gums, a sinking but slightly rapid pulse, and a red, dry tongue, she was put on Isatis Cooling (5 tablets TID) and Quiet Digestion (2 tablets every

2 hours). I also suggested she start on Colostroplex (1 tablet TID), increasing or decreasing the dosage as necessary. After three weeks, she reported a lessening of abdominal pain and tiredness, so I replaced Isatis Cooling with Phellostatin (2 tablets TID), which has more tonifying properties, and told her to take Quiet Digestion before meals. Two months later, she reported her bowel movements were normal, though she had two flare-ups, which were controlled by taking Isatis Cooling and Quiet Digestion every 2 hours thereafter. Her overall energy had improved, and she seemed to recover from flare-ups more quickly. She will use the Digestive Clearing Diet to identify problem foods.

Case #5
Rafael, 35, had been to almost ten doctors by the time I saw him. His main symptom was abdominal cramping, which was so severe that he "felt like a brick" was in his right lower abdomen. Although he had undergone countless medical tests to rule out Crohn's disease and other gastrointestinal complaints, his final diagnosis was IBS. His medical doctors advised him to increase his fiber and liquid intake, and suggested a bulking agent. He was also prescribed an antidepressant, which initially helped reduce the intestinal spasms, but after a year it began losing its effectiveness and he was experiencing side effects.

He told me during our consultation that his gastrointestinal symptoms had started ten years ago following a trip to South America where he contracted amoebic dysentery and was put on Flagyl. Traditional Chinese diagnosis revealed that his pulse was sinking and rapid, his tongue slightly red. Because many parasites are Flagyl-resistant, I suggested trying the antiparasitic formulas Artestatin and Aquilaria 22 (1 tablet of each TID). I also recommended peppermint and passionflower tea (3 cups per day) to ease his nerves, and to help relieve the cramping, Quiet Digestion (1 to 2 tablets as needed) was to be chewed.

As he gained control over his nerves, he walked to the gym a few times a week to play racquetball. He experienced one flare-up, for which he was given Isatis Cooling in bulk herb form; he later indicated that it was effective in saving him a trip to the emergency room. During the following six months on the above herbal protocol, his various symptoms were either eliminated or greatly reduced. Quiet Digestion nearly always resolved his acute symptoms.

Case #6

Sylvie, an overweight woman in her 40s, had a medical diagnosis of IBS. She complained of constant diarrhea, which had to be controlled by Lomotil; her other symptoms were abdominal cramping and general nervousness and irritability. Her diet journal revealed that she was eating cheese or yogurt several times per day. She also drank diet sodas and several cups of coffee. I explained that Chinese medicine considers dairy foods as damp and heat producing and that she would be better off eating lean meat as a protein source. Traditional Chinese diagnosis revealed that her pulse was slow and soggy, and tongue pale and red on the edge. I recommended Woman's Balance (2 tablets TID) to promote energy circulation and suggested Colostroplex (1 tablet TID) for diarrhea. On a telephone follow-up, she said that the diarrhea was better, but that she was not able to make any dietary modifications or engage in daily exercise. She canceled her next appointment.

Case #7

Yvonne, 45, is a computer graphics professional. She was diagnosed with IBS. Her main symptoms were tiny bowel movements that required straining, followed by an urgent need to defecate five minutes later. She also experienced gas and bloating. Yvonne reported feeling tired and "toxic," as well as constantly cold. Her symptoms had been going on for ten years, following a divorce. During this period she worked at a job that she disliked and was going to night school. She admitted to having difficulty expressing her emotions. Traditional Chinese diagnosis found that her pulse was wiry, and her tongue had a thick white coating.

I advised Yvonne to undertake a stress reduction program, to exercise every day, and to use positive affirmations. I recommended an herbal decoction consisting of herbs for moving liver Qi and strengthening the spleen, as well as the formulas Heavenly Water (2 tablets TID) and Quiet Digestion (1 tablet before meals and 1 to 2 tablets as needed) to relieve gas. I also counseled her to eat four to five small meals per day instead of three large ones. One month later, she had enrolled in a yoga class and was practicing yoga every day for half an hour. She was also eliminating dairy products. Her tongue coating was now normal and her pulse was less wiry. We discontinued the bulk herbs and she began taking Six Gentlemen (2 tablets TID) while continuing with Heavenly Water. She also took Quiet Digestion before and after meals. All symptoms were improved after two months.

Case #8
Lois, a 48-year-old lifetime smoker, came in with IBS. Her main symptoms were constipation, gas, intestinal cramping, chronic sinus problems, and frequent colds and flus. She developed a cold or flu after each time she traveled by plane, which was often since her extended family lived all over the country. Traditional Chinese diagnosis found that her pulse was sinking, though fast, her tongue red, cracked, and had a grayish coating, all of which, in addition to her greenish sputum, indicated heat. I recommended a thermos of peppermint tea for gas and cramping, and 1 teaspoon of flax seeds daily for constipation. Nasal Tabs (2 tablets QID), which contains rhubarb to help move the bowels, and Coptis Purge Fire (2 tablets QID) to resolve damp-heat were recommended.

After two weeks, her sinuses were only slightly congested, her tongue appeared less red and the coating returned to normal, therefore I recommended that she discontinue the Coptis Purge Fire. Although she experienced less straining, she still had difficulty in moving her bowels, so Gentle Senna formula (3 tablets at bedtime) was added. To alleviate the persistent nasal congestion, I instructed her to use a eucalyptus oil steam by placing a few drops of eucalyptus essential oil in a pot of water, covering her head with a towel and breathing deeply through each nostril. I cautioned her that when using this treatment to be careful not to scald herself.

After four months of taking Nasal Tabs, Gentle Senna, peppermint tea, and flax seeds, all her symptoms were 90 percent improved. At this point she took Astra C (2 tablets TID) to build up her defenses and prevent colds and sinus problems, and continued taking peppermint tea and Gentle Senna as needed.

Indigestion

Indigestion is a term covering many symptoms commonly experienced after eating, such as discomfort caused by a feeling of fullness in the upper abdomen, heartburn, nausea, and bloating. Indigestion is a symptom, not a disease in itself. Almost everyone has occasional indigestion, but chronic indigestion can signal diseases such as peptic ulcer, gastritis, gastric cancer, or gallbladder disease. Alcohol, coffee, fried foods, and cigarettes can all contribute to, or cause, indigestion. Stress can be another factor. Some individuals also have sensitivity to specific foods that normally might not bother other people; such sensitivity can lead to indigestion. Discomfort while eating can be related to esophagitis or gastritis, while pain several hours after eating can point to duodenal ulcer or gallbladder disease. Your health professional may want to screen for blood in your stool or conduct other diagnostic tests to rule out other more serious conditions.

Antacids are the common conventional treatment, including drugs such as Tagamet (cimetidine) and Zantac (ranitidine). Such treatment is based on the common misconception, even among medical professionals, that the pain of indigestion is due to excess stomach acid. Clinical trials in the early 1990s demonstrated that antacids were of no benefit for the majority of subjects with "heartburn." Secretions from the pancreas, gallbladder, and small intestine normally neutralize any acid from the stomach that might reach the intestine, where it can cause pain. This neutralization occurs optimally only under conditions of rest, so eating in a hurry, eating while stressed or upset, or failing to relax after a meal may be the most common causes of indigestion pain. The problem is not excess acid, but rather not enough of the neutralizing secretions needed to counterbalance normal, or even low levels, of stomach acid entering the intestine.

Self Help

- Supplementation with acidophilus/bifidus/FOS products, mentioned in Chapter Three, help relieve indigestion. With heat signs, drink a cup of peppermint tea before meals; with cold signs, drink ginger with squeezed lime before meals
- Digestive Harmony (2 tablets TID or as needed) may be used

Professional Treatment

- Formulas such as Quiet Digestion (2 tablets TID to QID) can be administered; with cold signs, use Stomach Tabs (2 to 3 tablets TID)
- If indigestion is related to stress, Ease 2 (3 tablets TID) can be administered for loose stools, and Ease Plus (3 tablets TID)

for constipation. For strongest results combine with Quiet Digestion

Case Studies

Case #1

Delilah, a woman in her mid-60s, was affected by indigestion, a constant foamy phlegm in her throat each morning, and by afternoon coughing. Traditional Chinese diagnosis found that her pulse was sinking and fast, and her tongue had a thick white coating. I recommended that she eliminate all dairy and citrus products, especially orange juice. The first week, she was given Quiet Digestion (1 tablet every 2 hours). The next week, the dosage of Quiet Digestion was altered (2 tablets QID), and the formula Clear Phlegm (1 tablet QID) was introduced. After two weeks, her symptoms were 50 percent better. Later, after I inquired about her lifestyle habits, she admitted that she had beer a few times a week with her husband, although during her initial consultation she claimed that she was not a drinker. I advised her to give up beer. At her next visit, she reported that the indigestion was almost relieved, except when she drank beer or ate late at night.

Case #2

Annie, 81, suffered nausea, diarrhea, stomach cramps, and was on several medications. Other complaints included dry skin, constant thirst, and abdominal bloating. Traditional Chinese diagnosis revealed that she had a wiry, deficient pulse, and a swollen, dry, and cracked tongue. I suggested Quiet Digestion (2 tablets TID), which helped the diarrhea. After three weeks of herbs, the stomach cramps and nausea were much improved. She remained on Quiet Digestion while Woman's Balance (2 tablets TID) was added. After two more weeks, she reported all symptoms were nearly alleviated.

Case #3

Greta, 40, had pulmonary fibrosis and was awaiting a lung transplant. She was on oxygen and prednisone, and was experiencing excess acidity in her stomach. Traditional Chinese diagnosis found that her pulse was slippery, and tongue pale with a grey coating. I recommended Ease Plus (2 tablets QID) and Stomach Tabs (2 tablets QID). After two weeks, the herbs completely eliminated her indigestion, burping, and acidity.

Intestinal Obstruction

Intestinal obstruction is the partial or complete blockage of either the small intestine or the colon. Common symptoms include abdominal distention, spasms or cramping of the mid-abdomen, vomiting, and the inability to pass feces or intestinal gas. Partial obstruction may stimulate the intestines to secrete fluid, resulting in diarrhea. The abdomen may become swollen as a result of trapped intestinal gas and fluid. Intestinal obstruction can be due to scar tissue from previous operations, hernia, or a knotted, twisted intestine known as volvulus. Cancer is another cause, as is adynamic ileus, the failure of the intestines to transport food matter. Food allergies and intolerances can also lead to obstruction-like symptoms. Although a skilled herbalist can clear some obstructions, it is wise to consult with your physician in order to assess the risk of waiting for alternative methods to take effect, since obstruction can lead to life-threatening conditions, such as perforation of the intestines or even gangrene. Medical tests, such as X-ray, sigmoidoscopy, or colonoscopy, are conducted to assess the location of the obstruction. Sometimes these procedures actually relieve the obstruction. If they do not, a tube may be inserted through the nose to remove intestinal secretions and air from the small bowel. This is known as nasogastric suction. If the procedure is not successful, an operation may be necessary.

Case Study

Ruben, a 30-year-old HIV-positive patient, showed signs of an obstruction, although all conventional tests were negative. His symptoms included weekly episodes of severe cramping, diarrhea, and vomiting. These bouts lasted several hours, resulting in terrible fatigue. Traditional Chinese diagnosis revealed that his pulse was sinking, weak, and rapid, and tongue pale with a thick white coating. We recommended an herbal tea to tonify the spleen (8 ounces per day), and the herbal formula Colostroplex (1 tablet per day). Colostroplex was administered for its immune strengthening properties; it also binds and removes toxins from the gastrointestinal system. After two months, Ruben found that the herbal tea formula along with the Colostroplex seemed to reduce the severity of his weekly attacks. His pulse was stronger, and his tongue coating was less thick. Follow-up therapy consisted of Source Qi formula (3 tablets TID) along with Colostroplex.

Lactose Intolerance

Lactose intolerance can cause abdominal cramping and bloating, diarrhea, and intestinal gas. It is especially common among people of African, Asian, or Mediterranean origin, but also affects about 20 percent of Caucasians. The condition occurs when the lining of the small intestine does not produce adequate amounts of the lactase enzyme. Lactase is necessary to digest lactose, the natural sugar in milk and dairy products. Low lactase levels may also be present in other intestinal disorders, viral or bacterial infection, and cystic fibrosis. Milk pre-treated with lactase is commercially available. Lactase is also available in pill form, or as a liquid that can be mixed into milk. Some individuals with intolerance or allergy to milk are sensitive to the milk protein—called casein—rather than the milk sugar. Some people find that cheese and yogurt do not give them symptoms, whereas milk does. Others find goat's milk more tolerable than cow's milk. Another alternative is to use soy or rice milk. Humans, particularly North Americans and Northern Europeans, are the only mammals that drink milk as adults. In fact, many proponents of natural therapies feel that milk is unnecessary for adults.

Professional Treatment

- Colostroplex (1 to 2 tablets per day) may be used long-term to treat mild dairy intolerance. However, it is necessary to eliminate all dairy products for sixty days, then reintroduce offending products on an occasional basis. Acidophilus/bifidus and FOS are also recommended

Malabsorption

The main signs and symptoms of malabsorption are weight loss, weakness, diarrhea, abdominal cramps, gas, and bloating. In addition, there may be excessive fat in the stool, causing it to float or to have a bad odor. Protein may also be lost in the stool, resulting in tissue wasting. Vitamins A, B12, D, E, K, and folic acid may all be deficient. Calcium, too, may be lost, leading to calcium oxalate urinary stones and demineralization of the bones.

Self Help

- Acidophilus/bifidus/FOS supplements (use as directed on the label)
- Digestive Harmony (2 tablets QID) aids in the treatment of malabsorption

Professional Treatment

- Protein, vitamin, and mineral therapy as needed
- Phellostatin (1 to 2 tablets TID), Colostroplex (1 to 4 tablets daily), and an anti-yeast diet may help reduce gas and bloating
- Use Quiet Digestion (2 tablets TID or as needed) symptomatically to reduce cramps, gas, and bloating
- For diarrhea without bloody stools and low or normal temperature use Source Qi (3 to 5 tablets TID)
- For diarrhea with bloody stools and elevated body temperature use Formula H (3 to 5 tablets TID) and Colostroplex (1 to 3 tablets TID)

Case Study

Herbert, 70, was undergoing chemotherapy and radiotherapy for cancer. His main symptoms were weight loss, diarrhea, abdominal cramps, and intestinal gas. His medical doctor had prescribed a multivitamin and mineral preparation. Herbert's daughter had recommended a digestive enzyme product, which was minimally effective. Traditional Chinese diagnosis revealed that his pulse was sinking and slow, and his tongue had a thick white coating. I recommended Source Qi (3 tablets TID) along with Quiet Digestion (2 tablets TID and whenever he had gas). Additionally, I suggested that he drink hot powdered ginger tea before

183

meals. Within two weeks he reported less diarrhea, cramping, and intestinal gas. I then recommended increasing the dosage of Source Qi (5 tablets TID), and staying on Quiet Digestion. As he found the powdered ginger too spicy, I suggested he use fresh ginger with squeezed lime before meals. After four weeks he experienced diarrhea only occasionally and his wife said his mood and energy level had improved substantially. He had even gained a few pounds.

Megacolon

Megacolon is a condition in which the colon becomes abnormally large or dilated. The disease may be congenital or acquired. The chief symptoms of megacolon are severe constipation and abdominal distention. The colon becomes greatly enlarged due to nerve damage in the colon or rectum. Megacolon due to congenital absence of nerve cells in the distal part of the colon is known as Hirschsprung's disease. Acquired megacolon is usually due to poor bowel habits and is especially common in mentally retarded or psychotic children. Toxic megacolon, a serious complication of ulcerative bowel diseases and amoebic colitis, is a medical emergency because of the possibility of rupture of the colon. Other causes of megacolon include spinal cord injury, Parkinson's disease, Chagas' disease (a parasitic disease) and medications such as narcotics. Conventional medical treatment of megacolon consists of enemas, laxatives, or surgery. And when the cause is medications, the dosages should be decreased. Congenital conditions are almost always more difficult to treat with natural remedies than acquired conditions. The suggestions listed under "Chronic Constipation" may be helpful.

Pancreatitis

Acute pancreatitis is defined as an attack that does not lead to permanent damage, whereas chronic pancreatitis, by definition, causes permanent damage, and is usually progressive and irreversible. This condition is usually the result of chronic alcoholism or gallbladder disease. Chronic alcohol abuse can cause the pancreatic enzymes to become prematurely activated: the enzymes start digesting the pancreas itself. In gallbladder disease, a gallstone moving toward the intestine can block the pancreatic duct. Pancreatitis is a common side effect in HIV patients taking the medications ddI or ddC. Symptoms of pancreatitis include severe abdominal pain that radiates to the back. The pain appears suddenly and is persistent. The abdomen is tender, and pain is often severe in the upper abdomen and less severe in the lower abdomen. Many patients experience nausea and vomiting, as well as sweating. Conventional medical treatment is to fast until the symptoms disappear.

Professional Treatment

- Administer Coptis Purge Fire (3 tablets, 4 to 6 times per day) when pancreatitis is accompanied by a thick, greasy tongue coating, jaundice, and fever. For pain, combine Coptis Purge Fire with GB-6 (2 tablets, 4 to 6 times per day) or Channel Flow (2 tablets, 4 to 6 times per day)
- GB-6 and Channel Flow (2 to 3 tablets, 4 to 6 times per day for each formula) are the primary formulas for addressing radiating pain, nausea, and vomiting that are unaccompanied by fever
- For fever without jaundice but with radiating pain, administer Clear Heat and Isatis Cooling (2 tablets of each formula, 4 to 6 times per day)

185

- Pancreatic enzymes may be used
- Acupuncture is useful for relieving acute pain (see Appendix C)

Parasites

Parasites are a growing problem in the developed countries due to an increase in air travel and water supplies infected by animal waste. Secondary factors are inadequate sterilization and poor hygiene practices at restaurants and day care centers, and drinking untreated water while hiking or camping. Common symptoms are digestive complaints that do not clear up, headache, fatigue, muscle aches, joint pain, propensity toward food and environmental sensitivities and allergies. If you have had a chronic digestive condition that has resisted treatment, and have traveled to Asia, South America, or Africa, it is very likely you have a parasitic condition. The same is true if you have consumed untreated water while camping or hiking. Unfortunately, many physicians in the U.S. are not aware of the rising incidence of parasite infections. Even as far back as 1976, the Centers for Disease Control (CDC) reported that one of every six people tested in the U.S. at random had one or more parasites.

One type of infection, giardiasis, is so common in some areas that almost the entire indigenous population host this microorganism. Also known as "Montezuma's Revenge" or "Delhi Belly," giardiasis can cause violent cramping and diarrhea that continues despite the use of over-the-counter remedies. *Giardia* organisms can be found in mountain streams, and more alarming is the fact that they can infect city water systems, since *Giardia* is not killed by chlorination. In day care centers *Giardia* and other parasites may be spread by direct contact with feces during diaper changing, as well as by children coming in contact with feces and then inserting their hands in their mouths, touching toys or drinking faucets, and engaging in other shared contact.

The immune-compromised are especially vulnerable to parasitic infections, including two in particular, toxoplasmosis, which is transmitted by cats, and cryptosporidiosis, which is acquired through drinking water.

Parasites can also be passed through sexual contact. Improper cooking and preparation of foods is another possible source of parasitic transmission. If you enjoy sushi, you should always eat at a reputable restaurant, where the chefs practice proper food preparation and sanitary habits, such as frequent hand washing.

Parasites can wreak havoc in the body. Some infections can be fatal if untreated. Parasites can destroy cells and produce toxic substances. They irritate the body's tissues, causing inflammatory reactions. Untreated infections result in the body's immune system producing too many specialized white cells, called eosinophils. Eosinphils can cause tissue damage as they multiply to wipe out the parasites, resulting in pain and inflammation. Also, the immune system becomes exhausted in its intense effort to battle parasitic infection.

Flagyl (metronidazole) is the most common drug used in the U.S. to treat parasites, but it has many side effects. Also, many parasites are Flagyl resistant.

What can you do if you have unrelieved digestive disorders or other strange symptoms that have remained untreatable, especially if you have been exposed to one of the above infection pathways? Find a holistic practitioner who can adequately diagnose parasites, or go to a university-affiliated hospital or clinic that has a department of parasitology or tropical medicine.

Preventing Parasites

+ Filter water. This is especially necessary for the immune-compromised and international travelers. Bottled water may not be pure, or bottles may not be properly sterilized. Take along a water sterilization kit (camping stores often provide information about which kits and filters are appropriate for your needs)

- Be careful about eating out. Eat only properly cooked foods when you are unsure of the cleanliness standards
- Vegetables and fruits should be peeled
- Make sure you have separate cutting surfaces for meats and vegetables. These areas should be pet free
- Have household employees tested for parasites
- Have pets checked on a regular basis for parasites
- Keep pets away from food preparation areas
- Never kiss pets or allow them to sleep with your family
- Protect children from animal droppings
- Immune-compromised persons should not handle cat litter. If this is not possible, use surgical gloves and wear a face mask, while keeping the litter as far away from the body as possible. Wash hands thoroughly afterward
- Practice safe sex

Chlorine food bath: Use ½ teaspoon of Clorox bleach to 1 gallon of water. Leafy vegetables, thin-skinned fruits, and all meats (separate baths for different meats) should be placed in the bath for 20 minutes. Then, place in clear water for 10 minutes. Thoroughly clean and dry all food treated this way. This procedure can be used by susceptible individuals, and those living in areas of known infestation.

Freezing: Freeze fish for 48 hours, beef and pork for 24 hours. This procedure will kill any larvae.

Cooking: Make sure meat is thoroughly cooked (no pink showing). When eating out, request that meat be cooked well done. At home, cook meat at a minimum of 325°F (162.7°C), fish at

400°F (204.4°C). Beef, lamb, veal, and pork should be cooked to an internal temperature of 170°F (76°C). Fish should be cooked at 140°F (60°C) for at least 5 minutes.

Professional Treatment

- Aquilaria 22 (1 to 3 tablets TID) plus Artestatin (start at 1 tablet per day, increase to 6 to 9 per day over a two week period) can be taken before meals
- With constipation, increase Aquilaria 22, decrease Artestatin dosages
- With diarrhea, increase Artestatin, decrease Aquilaria 22 dosages
- Use Quiet Digestion (2 tablets TID or as needed) for cramping, intestinal gas, and poor digestion
- Use Colostroplex (1 to 6 tablets per day) to help bind and eliminate toxins. Decrease dosage if constipation results
- After 3 months of Artestatin and Aquilaria 22, if parasites are still evident, consider Biocidin (use as directed) or black walnut hulls (start at 1 capsule, try to increase to 10 to 15 daily). I recommend these products be taken consecutively, not at the same time
- As an adjunct, 2 cloves of raw chopped or chewed garlic (not heated) can be taken. Garlic is considered effective for amoebic dysentery and other parasite infections. Note that prepared garlic formulas may not be effective for parasites, and some individuals are sensitive to garlic

Case Studies

Case #1
Doug, 50, suffered intense lower right quadrant pain and high fever once or twice a year, lasting four to seven days. These attacks began following a trip to China several years ago. Conventional

medical tests were negative for ulcers, parasites, and appendicitis. A chiropractor told him that he had a fungal infection of the ileo-cecal valve. Doug had a history of hepatitis, although his liver enzymes were not elevated. He had tried various herbal combinations for the pain, but the condition persisted. Traditional Chinese diagnosis found that his pulse was wiry, and his tongue flabby (revealing dampness) and red around edges, with a greasy coating.

I prescribed a general cleansing protocol that addressed both parasites and *Candida,* surmising that he had contracted a parasitic infection in China that was undiagnosable by Western tests. As the primary remedy, I recommended Aquilaria 22 (2 tablets TID, since his stools were normal) to be taken for three months. He was also given Artestatin (1 tablet TID) for two months, followed by Phellostatin (2 tablets TID) for one month. After two weeks, he reported some cramping, which he believed was due to the herbal formulas. I suggested that he reduce the dosage of Artestatin to 2 tablets a day, and if he still experienced cramping to reduce the dosage further (Artestatin is especially effective in killing amoebic cysts, however cramping is a sign that the dosage should be reduced). I indicated that he could also reduce the dosage of Aquilaria 22. Since I believed that he might have been having a die-off reaction, I started him on the preparation Ecliptex (2 tablets TID), which is useful for detoxifying the liver.

Two weeks later he developed a cold of the wind-cold variety, so I recommended Isatis Gold (3 tablets, 4 to 6 times per day) and told him to temporarily discontinue the antiparasitic herbs. As he was having loose stools, fatigue, and abdominal pain following the initial cold symptoms, I recommended Quiet Digestion and Ease 2 (2 tablets TID of each formula); the latter is a traditional remedy used to address lingering cold symptoms. He reported feeling better a few days later after using this protocol. He felt less achy, but still experienced some loose stools, so he continued on the formulas for a few more days. When he felt better, I advised him to resume the Aquilaria 22 (1 tablet TID) and Quiet Digestion (2 tablets TID) for a week before going back to the Artestatin. He continued to take the three remedies for a few more weeks. As he was about to go on a business trip and had no digestive symptoms, I recommended he continue to take the Aquilaria 22 (1 tablet TID), Artestatin (1 tablet per day), Ecliptex (2 tablets TID), and Quiet Digestion (as needed).

When he returned from his business trip, he reported that the Quiet Digestion had given him symptomatic relief on a few occasions. He asked my opinion about addressing the fungal infection and I indicated that Aquilaria 22 and Phellostatin had antifungal properties. His new regimen therefore was Aquilaria 22 (1 tablet TID), Phellostatin (1 tablet TID), Ecliptex (2 tablets TID), and Quiet Digestion (as needed).

A few weeks later, Doug contracted food poisoning. I told him to take Quiet Digestion (2 tablets, 4 to 6 times per day) and to chew 1 tablet of Aquilaria 22 every few hours. He reported great relief. He remained on a maintenance protocol of Aquilaria 22 (1 tablet TID), Phellostatin (1 tablet TID), and Ecliptex (2 tablets TID) for another month. As of this writing, he has not had an episode of appendicitis-like pain in one year. He uses Quiet Digestion symptomatically for digestive upset.

Discussion: Doug's case demonstrates that antiparasitic formulas should be administered long-term for best results. Also, those who have parasitic infections are more susceptible to colds, the flu, and food poisoning. Finally, it is not uncommon to have parasitic and fungal infections simultaneously.

Case #2
Samantha is a health professional who developed chronic diarrhea after a vacation to Mexico four years ago. Following a thorough biomedical evaluation, she was treated with Flagyl. However, she continued having up to ten episodes of watery

stools per day. She also suffered from fatigue, occasional headaches, and joint pain. Traditional Chinese diagnosis found that her pulse was weak and slow, and tongue pale and swollen. I recommended a combination of Source Qi formula (3 tablets TID for the first week, 5 tablets TID thereafter), along with an herbal antiparasitic, Artestatin (1 tablet TID). The first week, she reported cramps after taking the herbs, so I suggested reducing the dosage of Artestatin to 1 tablet per day and maintaining the Source Qi dosage (3 tablets TID). By the end of the second week, her stools were more formed, but the frequency—especially in the morning— was unchanged. At this point, Colostroplex (1 tablet TID) was added to the existing protocol. At the end of the fourth week, the urgency and number of stools had decreased. She was referred to a lab specializing in parasitic diseases, where they found the presence of *Histoplasma capsulatum,* a fungus. Therefore, I suggested increasing the dosage of Artestatin 2 tablets per day, as well as taking the herbal antifungal Biocidin (2 drops on a cracker with meals). She also continued taking Colostroplex (1 tablet TID) and Source Qi (3 tablets TID).

At the end of the third month, her stools were mostly normal, with an occasional bout of watery stools. The joint pain and headaches had disappeared. She continues to take the herbs until all symptoms are alleviated and parasite tests are negative.

Peptic Ulcers

Peptic ulcers are raw areas affecting either the stomach or the upper part of the small intestine. The stomach lining produces hydrochloric acid and a digestive enzyme called pepsinogen to aid in the digestive process. Once pepsinogen is secreted into the acidic environment of the stomach, it is converted into pepsin, a powerful enzyme that breaks down proteins. The stomach and upper intestine have specialized linings, which normally resist digestion by acid or pepsin. When the protective factors in the stomach and intestinal linings are deficient, and pepsin and acid damage the tissues of the lining, peptic ulcers result. These ulcers are similar to mouth ulcers (canker sores). A burning pain or gnawing ache is felt just below the breastbone when acid invades the raw ulcers. Ulcers in the stomach are called gastric ulcers, and those in the first part of the small intestine, duodenal ulcers. Eating food helps coat the stomach and temporarily relieve symptoms. Frequently, ulcer pain occurs at night, sometimes waking up the sufferer.

Ulcers can have serious consequences, especially perforation, when the ulcer penetrates all the way through the organ wall into the abdominal cavity, which can have fatal consequences. Ulcers can also cause internal bleeding into the digestive tract. One sign of this is black, tarry stools.

Lifestyle factors are associated with ulcers, especially smoking, drinking alcohol, and excessive stress. These probably cause a weakening of the stomach or duodenal lining. Taking anti-inflammatory medication, such as aspirin and other pain medications can also break down the mucosal lining. About 2 to 4 percent of people taking such medications regularly develop bleeding ulcers and require hospitalization.

Scientists have recently acknowledged that a bacterium known as *Helicobacter pylori* can cause mucosal damage, stomach inflammation (gastritis), and peptic ulceration. *Helicobacter* infection is present in as many as 80 percent of ulcer cases, and is now recognized as a major cause of weakening of the mucosal lining, leading to ulcers.

Other factors, especially excess protein and fat in the diet, increase the secretion of stomach acid and slow the digestive process. This increases the exposure of the mucosa to the digestive enzymes. Some individuals naturally produce more stomach acid and are therefore more prone to ulcers.

Powerful antacids that shut off the secretion of acid by the stomach are the most powerful treatment for acute ulcers, allowing them time to heal. Antibiotics such as Flagyl (metronidazole), Prilosec (omeprazole), and Prevacid (lansoprazole), as well as bismuth products (such as Pepto Bismol®) have been added to the regimen when infection with *Helicobacter pylori* is diagnosed. Antacid treatment is valuable for the healing of ulcers, but without removing the underlying cause, recurrences are common. In fact, recurrences are more frequent in patients treated with drugs than in patients whose ulcers are allowed to heal on their own.

Patients who have burning pain, belching, and bloating, and do not show ulceration according to X-ray or endoscopy, are considered to have dyspepsia, resulting from a low grade stomach or duodenal inflammation.

Self Help

- Cruciferous vegetables, especially cabbage, fenugreek seeds, figs, and ginger or licorice tea (ginger is contraindicated in a heat pattern, licorice tea in cases of high blood pressure) strengthen the stomach lining so that it is less likely to be eaten away by acids. These foods also trigger the release of mucus, which covers the stomach cells with a protective coating
- Avoid milk and dairy products. Milk is no longer thought to be effective in helping ulcer patients, and may actually be harmful since protein rich foods and calcium may stimulate acid production

Professional Treatment

- For burning pain, use Isatis Cooling (3 tablets TID to QID), which also has antibacterial and antiviral properties
- For concomitant indigestion, combine Isatis Cooling with Quiet Digestion (2 tablets TID to QID)
- For stress, use Ease Plus (3 tablets TID), a beneficial antacid remedy
- For cold signs, use Stomach Tabs (3 tablets TID)

Case Studies

Case #1

Arthur, a 40-year-old insurance agent, was diagnosed with *H. pylori* by his gastroenterologist. His main symptoms were gastric burning, indigestion, and occasional headaches. Because Arthur is very sensitive to antibiotics, he wanted a more natural therapy, so he decided to try herbs first. Traditional Chinese diagnosis found that his pulse was rapid and choppy, and tongue red with a yellow coating. I recommended Isatis Cooling formula (3 tablets TID), as well as Quiet Digestion (1 tablet before and after meals). I also suggested reducing or eliminating dairy products, soft drinks and citrus drinks, and that he take up walking after meals. He was already reducing his fat intake. Within two weeks, his condition was 50 percent improved, and within a month, 90 percent.

Case #2

Giovanni, a 50-year-old smoker, was 40 pounds overweight. His chief complaint was gastric ulcers. However, he also had mild hypertension, and was on Elavil (amitriptyline) and Prozac (fluoxetine) for depression. Traditional Chinese diagnosis found that his pulse was rapid, and tongue dry with a yellow coating. I recommended Quiet Digestion and Ease Plus (2 tablets QID of each

195

formula). I suggested he stop drinking cold beverages and follow the Digestive Clearing Plan. After two weeks, he reported significantly less indigestion. He had stopped drinking iced beverages, but felt too stressed to make any other dietary changes.

Case #3

Arleen, a 24-year-old secretary, had a history of ulcers, carpal tunnel syndrome, severe menstrual cramps, and PMS. Her first ulcer was diagnosed at age 18, and she was treated with the drug Zantac (ranitidine). Her second episode with stomach discomfort occurred when she was 20 and under great emotional stress. Her gastroenterologist felt that she did not have an ulcer, and referred her to a psychiatrist. When I saw her, the gastrointestinal discomfort was secondary to the other symptoms. In Chinese medicine, all of the abovementioned symptoms and conditions are related to liver Qi stagnation. Her pulse was wiry, and tongue purple. The primary treatment for Arleen involved using SPZM (3 tablets TID) and Resinall K (½ dropper TID, as well as topically for carpal tunnel symptoms). After two weeks she reported the herbs to be helpful. At this point she was beginning to have signs of PMS, so the herbal protocol was adjusted to include Woman's Balance (2 tablets TID) and SPZM (3 tablets TID), and she continued to apply the Resinall K topically.

Case #4

Tony, a thin 44-year-old male, tested positive for *H. pylori*. His medical doctor prescribed tetracycline, Flagyl, and Pepto Bismol, which were 50 percent helpful in relieving the symptoms. But the drugs also caused side effects, including stomach cramping, abdominal burning, and fatigue. Traditional Chinese diagnosis found that he had a fast, wiry pulse, and a gray tongue coating. I recommended Isatis Cooling and Quiet Digestion (2 tablets TID of each formula) for two weeks following the drug therapy.

Isatis Cooling contains antibacterial herbs as well as herbs that promote circulation. Quiet Digestion addresses digestive symptoms. Only mild progress was seen after three weeks, so Channel Flow, a pain relieving formula, was added. He was thus taking Isatis Cooling, Quiet Digestion, and Channel Flow (2 tablets TID of each formula). After two weeks he said that he was 90 percent improved. Since I believed that stress was a contributing factor to his ulcers, I had him follow up with a combination of Ease Plus and Calm Spirit (2 tablets QID of each formula) to help him feel more relaxed.

Rectal Itching and Burning

Rectal itching, also known as *pruritis ani,* can have many causes, including dermatological disorders such as psoriasis, allergic reactions to food or medications, fungal and bacterial infections, and poor hygiene. Some foods, such as caffeine, nuts, chocolate, and chili peppers have also been implicated. It is important to determine the cause in order to establish proper treatment. Poor hygiene and food allergies must be eliminated. Dermatological disorders are treated with specific herbal teas or tablets. An anti-*Candida* diet can also be considered, in conjunction with Phellostatin (1 to 2 tablets TID).

Reflux Esophagitis (See also "Indigestion")

This disorder may be experienced as a sour taste in the mouth and can involve burning pain in the upper abdomen and mid-chest. The acidic contents of the stomach flow back into the esophagus, causing inflammation. While eating too quickly will bring this about occasionally for some, for others it is a chronic problem. Normally, the lower esophageal sphincter (LES) prevents the acidic contents of the stomach from moving upward into the esophagus. During swallowing, the LES is relaxed. If the LES relaxes at other times, however, heartburn occurs. X-rays and an endoscopy will help confirm the diagnosis.

Self Help

Two important ways of relieving reflux esophagitis are to elevate your head while sleeping, and to avoid bending over after eating, since this encourages reflux into the esophagus. In addition, eat slowly, stop smoking, lose weight, and avoid tight-fitting clothing, which can restrict circulation. Acidic foods—particularly chocolates, alcohol, citrus juices, and coffee—as well as fatty foods should be avoided. Late night snacks, heavy meals, or lying down after meals can exacerbate this condition. If you experience difficulty swallowing, or it feels like food is getting stuck on the way down, see your physician as soon as possible, since these signs may signal stricture formation or esophageal cancer.

Professional Treatment

- Ease Plus (2 tablets QID) is used to reduce heat as well as correct the counterflow of Qi
- Quiet Digestion (2 tablets QID) is used to encourage the movement of food through the digestive system; this formula can be combined with Ease Plus
- Stomach Tabs (3 tablets QID) is used to address cold signs

Case Studies

Case #1
Larry, a 54-year-old physician, complained of reflux esophagitis and insomnia. He was overweight by about 30 pounds and on

the drug Prilosec (omeprazole), which he wanted to stop. He was also on thyroid medication, which greatly helped his fatigue. Traditional Chinese diagnosis found that his pulse was weak and slippery, tongue pale with a greasy coating; he appeared tired and exhausted. I recommended Ease Plus and Quiet Digestion (2 tablets QID of each formula). In addition, I recommended at least 3 cups a day of peppermint or chamomile tea and at least 32 ounces per day of water. I also suggested that he participate in competitive sports to increase his metabolism and raise the Yang, in terms of Chinese medicine.

Two weeks later, there was no improvement. It turned out that he had taken the prescribed herbs only twice daily instead of four times per day as suggested, nor had he used the tea. As his insomnia was particularly severe, I also recommended that he start on the formula Schizandra Dreams (3 to 5 tablets at bedtime). After one month on the herbs and teas as recommended, he began tapering off the Prilosec, as all symptoms were reduced.

Case #2
Gloria, 42, was about 100 pounds overweight. She complained of chronic abdominal bloating, heartburn, and belching. Traditional Chinese diagnosis found that her pulse was sinking and wiry, and tongue red with a yellow coating. I suggested the formula Quiet Digestion (2 tablets QID). I explained to Gloria that the herbal remedies would have a minimal effect unless she changed her diet and got more exercise, such as walking every day, in addition to playing tennis with her daughter whenever possible. I also suggested increasing her consumption of whole foods, such as fresh fruits and vegetables and whole grains. I did not support any radical dieting, as it would only lead to feelings of deprivation and then binging, which she admitted was a problem for her. I advised she substitute herbal teas for sodas.

After two weeks she reported that her heartburn had

diminished, but the bloating and belching were still present. GB-6, a gallbladder formula that addresses food stagnation, was added (2 tablets TID on an empty stomach). She continued with Quiet Digestion with a slight change in dosage (1 tablet before and after each meal). I told her if she did binge, the Quiet Digestion would help her feel better the next day, as she admitted that she ate like how "an alcoholic drinks." She would feel hungover from "eating sweets," experiencing fatigue, difficulty thinking clearly, and abdominal aching. She would then eat more to feel better. Two weeks later, Gloria indicated that she believed the GB-6 was aggravating her digestion, so I suggested that she reduce the dosage. She also complained that she hadn't lost any weight, an indication that she hadn't made any of the dietary changes. Herbs have limited effects, unless they are combined with dietary modification, stress reduction, and an exercise program.

Scleroderma

Scleroderma is an autoimmune connective tissue disorder. It results in thickening and tightening of the skin, causing loss of flexibility, puffy hands and feet, and joint pain and stiffness. Scleroderma can also affect the esophagus and cause heartburn, and when the intestine is involved, both the absorption of nutrients and intestinal motility are impaired. Diarrhea can result from bacteria overgrowth.

Professional Treatment

- To treat connective tissue disorders herbs such as ginkgo and those rich in bioflavonoids are often used, or formulas containing ginkgo such as Flavonex (3 tablets TID) can be administered

- For poor intestinal motility and bacterial overgrowth, Colostroplex (1 to 2 tablets BID) and acidophilus/bifidus/FOS are recommended
- Herbal formulas, such as Mobility 2 (3 tablets QID), based on Clematis and Stephania herbal formula, are used to treat joint pain and puffy hands and feet. If joint pain worsens in cold, damp weather, consider Mobility 3 (3 tablets QID)

Case Study

Cherelle, a 39-year-old African American woman, came to our clinic with a medical diagnosis of scleroderma and colon problems suspected of being Crohn's disease. Her particular complaints were arthritis in the knees, left abdominal pain, and feeling like she wanted to go to the bathroom but couldn't. Traditional Chinese diagnosis revealed that her pulse was fast, and tongue red. She was given an herbal decoction similar to Mobility 2 and Clear Heat to clear toxins, tonify the kidney, and eliminate pain. After one week on the decoction, Cherelle reported more energy, a gradual reduction of pain, and less urgency to go to the bathroom. For the first time in a year she felt as though she could resume working. To follow up, it was suggested that she take Sea-Q (sea cucumber; 1 tablet BID) and Mobility 3 along with Six Gentlemen (2 to 3 tablets QID of each formula).

Short Bowel Syndrome

Short bowel syndrome is the result of surgery that removes significant portions of the small intestine, resulting in malabsorption problems. Pain and other symptoms still remain. Specific digestive formulas such as Quiet Digestion and pain relieving formulas such as Isatis Cooling may be used, as well as routine treatments for *Candida* and food intolerance.

Swallowing Problems

Regurgitation of food, chest discomfort while swallowing, gurgling sounds, or food or liquid stuck in the throat or esophagus can be a sign of swallowing problems. If you have difficulty or pain on swallowing, you should seek medical advice. Swallowing problems can be associated with serious diseases such as myasthenia gravis and esophageal cancer. Complete blockage is a medical emergency requiring immediate attention.

Globus is a feeling of having a lump in the throat without having any actual problem swallowing food. Stress is thought to be a main trigger. Other swallowing problems, such as achalasia, diffuse spasm, pharyngeal diverticula, pharyngeal paralysis, and esophageal stricture are more severe conditions and may require surgery. If surgery is not necessary, Chinese herbal medicine can be very effective for this condition. In Chinese medicine globus is known as "plum pit Qi," meaning one has the sensation that a plum pit is stuck in the throat.

Professional Treatment

- Stomach Tabs (3 tablets TID) based on the traditional formula Pinellia and Magnolia Bark Decoction *(Ban Xia Hou Po Tang),* can be very helpful by itself or combined with Clear Phlegm *(Wen Dan Tang)* to resolve phlegm (2 tablets QID of each formula)

Tropical Sprue

Tropical sprue is a condition characterized by a sore tongue, diarrhea, weight loss, and anemia, affecting those who are from or visit the tropics. Symptoms may appear either soon or years after a person has left the tropics. Possible causes are bacterial, viral, or parasitic infection, vitamin deficiency (folic acid) or toxins found in rancid fats. Standard treatment usually consists of folic acid, vitamin supplements and antibiotics.

Professional Treatment

- Colostroplex (1 to 3 tablets TID) helps stop diarrhea and weight loss
- Quiet Digestion (2 tablets TID) can be used for gastric upset
- Phellostatin (1 to 2 tablets TID) is useful for candidiasis
- Aquilaria 22 (2 to 3 tablets TID) and Artestatin (1 to 3 tablets TID) can be administered for parasitic infections
- Astra Isatis (2 to 4 tablets TID) is effective for chronic viral or bacterial infection

Viral and Bacterial Infections

Viral infections of the gastrointestinal tract may cause watery diarrhea, abdominal cramping and pain, low grade fever, nausea, vomiting, aching muscles, and headaches. If you have bloody diarrhea or profuse diarrhea to the point of lightheadedness, seek medical attention immediately. Usually viruses are transmitted through infected food or water. The Centers for Disease Control (CDC) estimates that there are twenty-five million cases of GI infections, causing about 10,000 deaths in the U.S. each year. Antibiotics are not effective for viral illness. Anti-diarrhea drugs are not recommended, because they may interfere with elimination of the virus through the feces.

One of the most common viruses is the *rotavirus,* especially in children under 2 years old. It is often spread among children attending day care centers and seniors in nursing homes. Rotavirus infections usually occur in the winter. It has an incubation period of one to three days. The typical symptoms are watery diarrhea, vomiting, and low-grade fever lasting five to eight days.

The *Norwalk virus* is usually found in contaminated food or water, causes gastroenteritis; the condition is also known as "winter vomiting disease." Diarrhea, nausea, and muscle ache may also be present. Outbreaks occur in families and communities, particularly among teenagers and adults. The time between the intake of contaminated food or water and the onset of symptoms ranges from four to seventy-two hours.

Campylobacter infections affect mostly children and young adults, and occur in the summer and fall. The cause is usually food, particularly milk and poultry, contaminated by this bacteria. The incubation period is two to four days. Symptoms include abdominal pain, nausea, low grade fever, headache, and muscle pain. The diarrhea is watery and can result in up to twenty bowel movements per day. The symptoms usually last less than a week, although relapses can occur. Antibiotics are usually recommended.

The *Salmonella* bacteria is perhaps the most widely known cause of food contamination. This organism is found in meats, poultry, eggs and egg products, non-pasteurized cheese, and milk, among other foods. Salmonella appears to occur more frequently in the meat of animals treated with antibiotics for growth promotion. Transmission is by fecal-oral contact (when, for example, you change a baby's diaper and do not wash your hands properly). The main symptoms are abdominal cramps, diarrhea, nausea, vomiting, and fever. Salmonella presents the greatest risk to infants and seniors. To prevent infection, food must be thawed properly and cooked adequately. Because antibiotic use prolongs the presence of the organism, such medications are not recommended unless localized infection (of the gallbladder, appendix, liver, or other sites) is suspected.

Shigellosis, or bacillary dysentery, is caused by the Shigella bacteria. This disease is very common in the developing world, and outbreaks occasionally occur in the U.S. Transmission is through fecal-oral contact, and is commonly spread by infected food handlers. The usual symptoms are cramping, abdominal pain, fever, and watery diarrhea that may contain blood and mucus. Conventional medical treatment involves rest and rehydration. Antibiotic use depends on severity of disease as well as age of the patient and possibility of further spread, among other considerations.

The *Escherichia coli (E. coli)* bacteria is normally found in the intestinal tract. The recent outbreaks of *E. coli* infection in the U.S. have raised a red flag over the food handling process, since this organism is primarily spread through the fecal-oral route. While the most common symptoms, GI upset and diarrhea, can be of concern, it is the more dangerous development of bacteremia (infection of the blood) that necessitates immediate medical intervention, since it can lead to septic shock and other life threatening complications. Conventional treatment therefore depends on the intensity of the symptoms. For diarrhea, treatment is rest and rehydration; for more severe symptoms, antibiotics such as trimethoprim-sulfamethoxazole, tetracycline, ampicillin, among others, may be used.

Anti-diarrheal medications should not be used, since they hinder the elimination of the bacteria. In all the above infections, if the symptoms are not so severe as to require a trip to your MD's office, time and the body's natural defenses are the greatest healers. In addition, the following remedies are helpful.

Professional Treatment

- Herbal formulas such as Isatis Gold (3 tablets QID, 4 to 6 times daily), which contain herbs such as isatis and goldenseal, are especially recommended. Isatis Gold has both antiviral and anti-bacterial properties
- Quiet Digestion (2 tablets TID to QID) helps speed up the removal of toxins; consider crushing two tablets and adding them to ginger tea if vomiting is present (see Chapter Three)
- For prolonged symptoms consider adding Ease 2 (2 to 3 tablets QID) to either Isatis Gold (2 to 3 tablets QID) or Quiet Digestion (2 to 3 tablets QID)
- Colostroplex (1 to 2 tablets TID) can be used after 1 to 2 days of infection; it stops diarrhea and has antiviral and antibacterial properties, and is thought to bind toxins and remove them through the gut. Acidophilus/bifidus and FOS may be helpful
- For side effects from antibiotics, Power Mushrooms (1 to 2 tablets TID) is used for cold signs as characterized by feeling cold, fatigue, or a lowered body temperature, sinking pulse and pale and/or coated tongue. If diarrhea accompanies cold signs, use Source Qi (3 to 5 tablets TID) instead. If signs of heat are present, such as elevated body temperature, add Phellostatin (2 tablets TID)

Other gastrointestinal infections, especially common in AIDS patients, include those due to cytomegalovirus and herpes simplex. The latter can cause anal pain, constipation, bloody diarrhea, and neurological symptoms such as thigh pain and numbness or tingling of the buttocks or anal area. The antiviral drug Zovirax (acyclovir) and analgesics are the standard conventional treatment.

Self Help

- Sitz baths may be beneficial (see Chapter Four)

Professional Treatment

- Astra Isatis (3 tablets TID) can prevent herpes; for cold signs add Power Mushrooms (1 to 2 tablets TID); for hot signs add Clear Heat (1 to 3 tablets TID)
- Colostroplex (1 to 2 tablets TID) is useful for bacterial and viral infections when diarrhea or loose stools are present
- Coptis Purge Fire (3 tablets, 4 to 6 times per day) is used for treating acute herpes outbreaks; reduce dosage if diarrhea occurs

Case Studies

Case #1

Claire, a 35-year-old athlete, had both chronic diarrhea and recurrent herpes simplex outbreaks. Traditional Chinese diagnosis found that she had a fast pulse, and red tongue. I recommended a combination of Colostroplex (2 tablets TID) and Astra Isatis (2 tablets TID). When outbreaks occurred she was to take Coptis Purge Fire (3 tablets, 4 to 6 time per day). Two months later she developed constipation, which frightened her, so I advised her to reduce the Colostroplex dosage to 1 tablet TID. Six months after starting the herbal formulas, she had only occasional diarrhea and the incidence of herpes outbreaks was reduced.

Case #2

Rodger, 42 and HIV-positive, experienced up to ten bowel movements a day. His other symptoms included fatigue, headaches, abdominal cramping, and retinitis caused by cytomegalovirus (CMV). His CD4 count was between 50 and 100. Rodger was being seen by several medical doctors specializing in HIV, and was taking AZT, antibiotics, and Foscavir for the retinitis. Traditional Chinese diagnosis found that his pulse was sinking and slightly rapid, his tongue was thin and dry with a coating on the edge.

I recommended Colostroplex (6 tablets per day) to reduce

diarrhea and Quiet Digestion (2 tablets as needed) to reduce abdominal cramping. After two weeks the diarrhea had in fact improved, so the dosage of Colostroplex was reduced (2 tablets BID). Quiet Digestion was partially effective in relieving abdominal cramps. At this point, he was advised to try Enhance (4 tablets QID), a formula shown in research to improve quality of life for HIV positive patients. After two months he was having normal bowel movements and experiencing less fatigue. He also believed that his eyesight was better, a phenomenon that I attribute to Colostroplex, which has apparently done the same for other individuals with CMV retinitis.

Whipple's Disease

Whipple's disease is a malabsorption syndrome found predominately in men over 40 years of age, causing symptoms such as diarrhea, abdominal pain, weight loss, low grade fever, and darkening of the skin. An unidentified organism is believed to be the cause. Diagnosis is made by biopsy of the small intestine. Long-term antibiotics are the usual medical treatment.

Professional Treatment

- Herbal formulas that have antiviral and antibiotic properties, such as Astra Isatis (3 tablets TID), can be administered
- Herbal remedies that support the digestive system, such as Six Gentlemen (3 tablets TID), are useful
- Colostroplex (1 to 2 tablets TID) may also be effective, especially for diarrhea

Zollinger-Ellison Syndrome

Zollinger-Ellison Syndrome is a rare digestive condition whereby tumors form in the pancreas or duodenum. The tumor secretes the hormone *gastrin,* which in turn promotes excessive acid secretion by the stomach. Up to 95 percent of those with this syndrome have peptic ulcers. The disease usually appears between ages 30 and 60. Up to 70 percent of those with Zollinger-Ellison Syndrome have malignant tumors that slowly spread to the lymph nodes and the liver. Ulcers associated with this syndrome are not easily treated with conventional ulcer medication or surgery. Surgery and medication such as Prilosec (omeprazole) are available. **Medical monitoring is very important with this disease.**

Professional Treatment

- Herbal formulas such as Cramp Bark Plus (3 tablets TID) may be useful in resolving tumors naturally. This formula has been used successfully in the treatment of uterine fibroids, however it must be used for six months or longer
- For stronger blood circulatory properties, combine Cramp Bark Plus with Regeneration (2 tablets of each QID)
- With fever and a heat pattern, use Unlocking with Crampbark Plus (2 tablets QID) of each formula
- Quiet Digestion (2 tablets TID) helps control acid if standard medication produces side effects

Chapter Notes

1. Jean Carper, *Food, Your Miracle Medicine* (New York: Harper Collins, 1993) 241.
2. Carper 43.
3. Ralph Golan, *Optimal Wellness* (New York: Ballantine Books, 1995) 377.

Chapter Five

◈

Digestive Clearing Diet

Digestive Clearing

If your goal is to greatly reduce or eliminate your digestive symptoms, you must be prepared to examine the foods you are eating. The terms "allergy," "intolerance," and "sensitivity," are used loosely by many people. A *food allergy* actually means that the body's immune system mounts a response to the offending allergen. A true allergy can be diagnosed by laboratory tests, such as with a skin prick, or radioallergosorbent test (RAST). Many persons with digestive disorders have *food sensitivities*, which cannot be detected by a laboratory test, but must be determined through trial and error. Sensitivities can cause such symptoms as abdominal cramping, diarrhea, constipation, intestinal gas, bloating, vomiting, nausea, ulcers, fatigue, joint pain, muscle aches, edema, headaches, migraines, depression, anxiety, respiratory difficulties, hyperactivity, and attention disorders.

Why are we so sensitive? We are exposed to thousands of chemicals our ancestors were never exposed to: pollutants, residues from fertilizer and pesticides, additives, preservatives, flavoring agents, among others. The earliest nutritionist was our nose and tongue. The foods we needed smelled good. When we had enough to eat, the food no longer appealed to our taste. With the advent of food processing, our senses of taste and smell were no longer reliable. And when the refrigerator and modern transportation came into being, foods that are genetically intolerable are now available.

Our ancestors ate what was available in their environments. The Native American Indian of the plains who was severely allergic to buffalo, the Asian who couldn't eat rice, or the Irish who couldn't eat potatoes, simply died. People then were much more active, so sensitivities were not taken into consideration. Everyday was a struggle for survival. When chased by wild animals, or fighting a warring tribe, one does not concern oneself about abdominal pain or constipation!

It is no wonder that millions of us have digestive disorders. We are bombarded with stress and don't exercise; we are exposed to foods and chemicals our digestive systems weren't designed to handle; and many of us were not breast-fed. Breastfeeding seems to protect us from developing allergies and sensitivities.

Another problem that people with digestive difficulties face is food cravings. Often, the cravings are for foods that one is actually sensitive to. I have counseled many digestive and respiratory patients who make statements like: "I must have cereal and milk every morning." Parts of the treatment involve refraining from the food one craves, in this case cereal and milk, for at least two weeks. Other unhealthy cravings may be dairy, alcohol, fruit, sweets, fructose, tomatoes, soy, and greasy foods. When the food cravings are based on emotional difficulties, psychological counseling may also be helpful.

You Can Heal

I have never met a person with a digestive disorder who has not been able to improve his or her condition with natural treatments. Does this mean that all these people are symptom free all the time? No, that would be unrealistic. What is realistic is that you can take some of the bite out of your digestive symptoms. In others words, you control your digestive system rather than letting it control you. Many clients have been able to reduce their symptoms so that they can lead more normal lives. Some of my clients have been able to avoid drastic surgeries, and others have been able to be weaned off strong pharmaceutical drugs that have debilitating side effects.

We live in an instant age with instant breakfast, instant banking, and computer dating; it's no wonder that we desire an instant cure. Rather than use a "Band-Aid approach," we can often obtain greater results by identifying the underlying cause of symptoms. Identifying the underlying reasons for the digestive disorder allows us to work on the root of the problem. Excess stress; eating foods we do not tolerate; and exposure to toxins such as bacteria, viruses, parasites, and fungi are often the basis for digestive problems.

The Digestive Clearing Program has helped thousands of people improve their digestive health. This program is suitable for most patients with chronic indigestion, ulcers, irritable bowel syndrome (IBS), acid reflux, heartburn, constipation, intestinal gas, diarrhea, diverticular disorders, Crohn's disease, ulcerative colitis, and gallbladder disease. We have found our program to be 90 percent effective for those who faithfully follow it. The program addresses exercise, stress reduction, and a change in diet. To facilitate your own digestive healing, I will ask you questions throughout the book to help you change how you think about food and your digestive problems. Although this is a self-treatment book, it is essential that you also see a health professional to get a thorough diagnosis. Your symptoms might be caused by something other than a digestive disorder, or you may have a rare condition that is not mentioned here, so please get a thorough biomedical evaluation. It is fine to show your health professional this book and to inform him or her about your decision to follow this program. Derivatives of this program are used in many clinics across the country.

By focusing on diet and the emotions, we can find the underlying cause of your symptoms. Even if you have inherited a gene that predisposes you to a digestive disorder, it is still possible through stress reduction and some diet detective work to overcome your condition. The treatment is to identify stressful emotions as well as discover which foods may be triggering symptoms in your body. If you think you may have come in contact with a toxin that is causing your digestive problem, it is essential that you see a health professional to be evaluated.

We will be focusing on stress-reduction techniques, exercise, and a specific way of eating that will help you evaluate your own food reactions. The program consists of a two-week preparation phase in which changes to your diet will be made gradually, followed by the two-week clearing phase. It is important to get daily exercise and do the stress-reduction techniques as specified. For best results, it is important that you follow the plan as stated. We recommend that you do twenty minutes of daily exercise. If walking twenty minutes per day sounds like too much, you may need to work up to this level before starting the program.

There are two stress-reduction techniques: meditation and abdominal massage. Certain experienced meditators may look at these techniques and think they are not advanced enough, but remember we are taking a vacation from our former lives. You can get back to your own routine at the end of the four weeks. Think of the four weeks as an experiment to regain your digestive health. It is important not to fight the program. Although at times you might get frustrated while undergoing the program, sabotaging it will only hurt you, as will trying to tweak the program by adding "just one little thing." The program is so powerful that some individuals find their digestive symptoms dramatically reduced in the first two weeks.

Sound good? Here are some of the people who have benefited from the program. Bob was a successful restaurant owner. Typically he worked twelve-hour days, six days a week. During work, he sampled delicious food, which was typically high in fat and calories. Bob also enjoyed wine and consumed several glasses daily. He was so busy managing his restaurant that he didn't have time to exercise. After turning 40, he noticed a persistent gut ache. Constant heartburn, sour belching, and constipation alternating with diarrhea were common. After seeing many medical doctors, he was diagnosed with gastroesophageal reflux disease (GERD). The doctors prescribed a strong stomach acid–blocking drug, which gave Bob headaches. At his wife's urging, he visited our clinic. He started the Digestive Clearing Program, and he took herbs to support his digestion. Bob noticed a significant improvement within three days. He learned several key points: (1) He had to balance work with quiet time, including exercise and meditation; (2) He had to limit his consumption of fatty foods; (3) When he sipped herbal teas throughout the day, he had more energy and less desire for coffee. Since he wasn't wired on caffeine, he didn't require alcohol to relax. The most difficult part of the program for Bob was eliminating alcohol for four weeks; however, his dramatic health improvement motivated him to limit alcohol consumption to weekends only. As long as Bob continues to take digestion-supporting herbs, exercises, and moderates what he eats, he doesn't have digestive problems.

Sue was a teacher, and although she had been a vegetarian for the past ten years, it was obvious that she wasn't healthy. She was overweight and had deep circles under her eyes. She was diagnosed with irritable bowel syndrome (IBS). Her doctor did not provide information about diet; he prescribed various muscle relaxants and medications for constipation and anxiety. The medications either produced significant side effects or didn't work. Sue needed coaxing to include fish in her diet. She started the Digestive Clearing Program, and after one week on the program she said she started to feel like her "old self." After completing the program and slowly reintroducing foods, she rarely had constipation or cramping and she lost twenty pounds. Sue learned that her body did not tolerate soy products or cheese.

Steve had coped with Crohn's disease his whole life and was hospitalized numerous times each year for severe pain. After following our digestive program, which included taking herbs and nutritional supplements, his life turned around in a major way. He was able to reduce his prescribed medications and was not hospitalized for almost a year. When he developed a form of arthritis called gout, he was prescribed a drug that almost immediately resulted in severe diarrhea. Although he was scared that he was having a flare-up of Crohn's disease, Steve reviewed his journal and realized that he had previously taken this same medication and that it had caused diarrhea. The diarrhea was not an exacerbation of his Crohn's disease, but a reaction to the medication he was taking. He notified his doctor and stopped the medication, and he was able to take a different medication that did not affect his digestion.

Chris's Case

Before starting the program, Chris reported constant gas, frequent cramping, and tiredness after eating. During the reintroduction phase, Chris identified three major problematic foods: milk, chocolate, and beans. Consequently, he avoided milk with cereal and ate chocolate or beans only when Digestive Harmony, an herbal blend, was on hand. He also discovered a sensitivity to excessive amounts of bread and pastries. Prior to the program, he ate bread or pastry with each meal. After the program, he ate one slice of bread per day. When he reduced or eliminated foods that his body didn't tolerate, his digestion improved, and he lost ten pounds. During the program, Chris also handled stress better; he learned to balance excess stress with activity, such as swimming. He found the abdominal massage (Chapter Four) invaluable to help expel gas. It made his whole body feel more comfortable.

After following the clearing program, aided by selected products, herbal teas, and a stress-reduction and exercise program, many clients are able to eat more freely than before.

Alan's Case

Alan was taking several pharmaceutical drugs, including anti-anxiety medications and acid blockers, and he complained of heartburn and constant bloating and gas pain. We used several techniques described in this book, including tuning into his symptoms and seeing if he could identify an emotion causing his symptoms. Once he found that he could make this connection, the discomfort was immediately reduced by 50 percent. Furthermore, he found that if he drank a cup of hot water with squeezed lemon or lime before meals and took Digestive Harmony, he did not have any digestive symptoms. This illustrates the power of combinations. Eventually he was able to eliminate all the drugs he was taking, with his doctor's approval.

Gail's Case

Gail was a 48 year-old woman who was very sensitive. After completing the program she found out that her body did not tolerate soy products or fruits. She also found that any food she ate daily seemed to compromise her digestive system, except for certain vegetables, chicken, and fish. To her surprise, she was symptom-free as long as she rotated her foods every day.

Program Overview

This program will help you identify problem foods. This is accomplished by eliminating foods that are difficult to digest and then reintroducing these foods after a two-week period. After reintroducing a food, symptoms will often return if you have a problem with the food in question. The advantage to this approach is that you will confirm which foods you do not tolerate well. You will take a break from foods that create havoc in your body. The program is designed to be a vacation for your digestive system. Similar to a vacation from work, it may not be pleasant 100 percent of the time, but it will be worth it in the long run. In addition, when you take more time to eat and minimize distractions, you can be in touch with your body's needs.

Program at a Glance

1. Prepare by reading this book. Consult with a health professional about beginning an exercise program. Review meal plans and recipes. Visit a health food store to stock up.
2. Weeks one and two are the introduction phase. Start moving toward a digestion-friendly diet. Eliminate fast foods, junk foods, wheat, dairy products, and soda. Dilute all fruit juices

by adding at least as much water as juice. All foods should be cooked. Drink sixty-four ounces of water or herbal tea each day. Keep a journal to log emotions, medications, and food reactions. Exercise to your level of stress and do daily stress-reduction for the duration of the program. Take Digestive Harmony and probiotics as directed. Digestive Harmony is based on a time-tested herbal digestive aid that promotes food absorption and alleviates symptoms of indigestion, gas, bloating, and mild cramping. A professional version, Quiet Digestion, is available through herbalists and other providers. Probiotics such as L–acidophilus are used to introduce healthy bacteria into the digestive tract, thus assisting the overall digestive process.

3. Weeks three and four are the clearing phase. Your diet will be low fat, moderate protein, with plenty of digestible vegetables and grains.

4. Week five begins the reintroduction phase. At this point add foods you have been avoiding in weeks three and four, in the recommended order.

Program Recommendations

During and after the program, it is important to drink at least 64 ounces of water or herbal tea daily. I recommend a cup of warm water with squeezed lemon or lime before each meal. Herbal teas such as peppermint, chamomile, ginger, or cinnamon will also aid digestion. Digestive Harmony is recommended with meals to further aid digestion. Take this product between meals if cramps, intestinal gas, or bloating are present.

Keeping a Journal

We suggest that you keep a journal before, during, and after the program so that you can identify any food-gut reactions, as well as to understand which emotions seem to trigger your digestive symptoms or make you more sensitive to foods. Very simply, you need to record the date, time, foods consumed, and any emotions experienced throughout the day, as well as the degree of discomfort. See if you can also add a cool thought. In other words, try to see if you can see the situation with greater balance. We suggest that you keep a pleasure log so that you chart your joy and happiness as well.

If you have any sensations, pleasant or unpleasant, it is important to see if you can attach an emotion, even if you are not sure what emotion you are feeling. Similarly, establishing a numerical value may not be possible, but it's important that you do the best you can. In terms of the cool thoughts, sometimes none may come to mind. If this is the case, just write "I'd prefer ... [describe the stressful or painful situation] was not happening, but I will handle it." One of my clients thought this was foolish, because he was convinced he was going to need an emergency surgery for one of his adhesions. "How can I handle it if I need to be rushed to the emergency room?" My reply: "Well, you'll handle it by going to the emergency room."

Food Emotional Journal

List the times you are eating, taking medication, or experiencing a strong emotion. To the right, write an assigned numerical value for the degree of discomfort, 0 being no discomfort, 10 being unbearable discomfort. When you have an uncomfortable feeling, do your best to describe the sensation: Are you angry, sad, overwhelmed, anxious, fearful, grief stricken? Underneath, be sure to list a cool thought; in other words, can you see your situation from a different perspective?

Time	Food	Event	Emotion	Degree of Discomfort *Scale of 1 to 10, 10 being the most discomfort, 0 being the least.*

Cool thought:

Pleasure Log

Any time you have a pleasant thought or experience joy or happiness, record it here. It is helpful to review your pleasure log any time you feel discouraged.

Time	Event or Pleasant feeling	Degree of Pleasure Scale of 1 to 7, 7 being the most pleasure, 1 being the least.

Tara's Case

Tara, a senior citizen, had a lifelong history of nervousness and symptoms of irritable bowel. Doctors told her to "live with it" or prescribed tranquilizers. In going over her journal, it became clear to her that she had too many commitments with her grown children (one of whom was disabled) her grandkids, her husband's business, her church duties, and a volunteer job she had reading to the blind. In addition, she located several food triggers. She found that as long as she cooked all her foods, minimized sweets, and stayed away from a green drink one of her friend's sold her, she did much better. She began to realize that she was happy on days she spent gardening and less happy with some of her other activities. She began to garden more, and before taking on a new project, she asked herself, *Do I really need to do this?* Her life satisfaction skyrocketed, and although she still has occasional symptoms, they do not bother her nearly as much as they used to. The following section is a sample from her journal. Jerry is her husband, and Kevin is her son, who lives at home.

Tara's Journal

2-1, 9 a.m.
Ate oatmeal, a little nervous about beginning of the program. Feeling nervous—8/10
Cool thought: It's always a little uncomfortable starting something new.

2-1, 10:30 a.m.
Felt violent cramps—tried to breathe deeply. Feeling disappointed—9/10
Cool thought: I think the breathing helped.

222

2-1, 10:35 a.m.
Jerry phoned, the bookkeeper called in sick, he wanted me to come in to work, but I promised Margie we'd go out for lunch. Now I don't know what do to. Feeling overwhelmed—10/10
Cool thought: Margie will understand. She always does.

2-1, 10:40 a.m.
Felt like I was going to throw up—actually had a dry heave. Why can't I call in sick? Frustrated—10/10
Cool thought: I didn't throw up.

2-1, 10:45 a.m.
Had another dry heave. That's it, I'm going to take a bath—I can't take a bath, it's 10:45 in the morning. What would my daughter say?—Take the bath—9/10
Cool thought: I can take a bath if I want to; they always help.

2-1, 11 a.m.
After bath—felt calmer—5/10
Cool thought: See, baths always help.

2-1, 11:05 a.m.
Called Margie and told her I was in no shape to go to lunch. She said she understood, such a great kid—grateful—3/10
Cool thought: I have a daughter who cares.

2-1, 12 noon
Tried to make myself eat, the food just didn't look too good, made myself a cup of tea and looked over *Healing Digestive Disorders*—2/10
Cool thought: At least I didn't force the food down.

2-1, 1 p.m.
Got to Jerry's business, made myself another cup of peppermint tea, felt better—1/10
Cool thought: Tea makes me feel better.

2-1, 3 p.m.

Got really panicky, then realized I hadn't eaten anything. Had a rice cake—3/10

Cool thought: Sometimes when I feel panicky it's just because I haven't eaten.

2-1 5 p.m.

Got stuck in traffic on the way home to make dinner, felt impatient—3/10

Cool thought: There's nothing I can do, so I won't worry about it.

2-1, 6 p.m.

Cooked spaghetti for Jerry and Kevin. I had a few bites of salad, then realized I wasn't supposed to have salad—Mad—6/10

Cool thought: I'm just going to have to stick it out and try the program. I had a baked potato; it tasted good!

2-1, 8 p.m.

Everything is calm in the house—calm—1/10

Cool thought: I'll do my stress-reduction exercise now while Jerry and Kevin watch TV.

2-1, 10 p.m.

Got hungry, had a rice cake—feel calm—1/10

Cool thought: I think the stress reduction helps.

Tara's Pleasure Log

2-1, 10 p.m.

Today was a good day. It was stressful, but I really think the stress reduction is helping. I did a good job—6/7

Deciding to Commit
to the Program

Radically improving your digestive health is simple, but not easy. Follow the Digestive Clearing Program for four weeks, get exercise and do stress reduction every day, and keep a journal to express your feelings and make note of your improvement. If you are reading this book, you probably want to improve your digestive health, but wanting to improve your digestive health and committing to follow the program are two different things. For example, millions of people each year want to quit smoking. Why are only a small number truly successful? Primarily because they have committed to a program. A program may include self-rewards for completion, support from others, and self-encouragement, which can be as simple as saying over and over, *I can do it; I'm doing a good job.* Finally, visualizing a future when you are in control of your digestive system helps a great deal.

With the Digestive Clearing Program you must decide whether it is truly important to change your digestive health. What do you want your life to be like? Visualize (or see in the mind's eye) what it would be like to have greater digestive health. Think of a reward you can give yourself when the four weeks are up. Who can support you when the going gets rough, a counselor, a priest, or a friend? What changes around food can you make in your personal and professional life?

Sally tried to do the program off and on for over one year. She noticed that she had fewer loose stools and cramping; however, her symptoms were not all gone. She had gone as far as three weeks into the program, when her food cravings became unbearable. She decided she had to have an ice cream sundae. Since she had already gone off the program, the following day she really pigged out on cookies and chips, and then her gut ached in a major way. Then she felt like a failure and ate more.

Another difficult aspect for Sally was exercise. She felt that she could do the program without the exercise; she had never liked exercise and was overweight and very self-conscious about exercise. What changed? Eventually Sally gave up trying to do the program and gained over 20 pounds, bringing her weight to over 200 pounds. Then her health insurance company told her that she would no longer be eligible for coverage because of her weight. Finally she decided that she had to do something. She made an appointment to see me. At my suggestion she took up walking, completed the first two weeks without a glitch, and rewarded herself by getting a massage the day after finishing her initial two weeks. Several important things happened: First, all her digestive symptoms went away; next, she lost 10 pounds; and then she had the self-mastery feeling that allowed her to continue with the reintroduction phase. *What strong reasons do you have for completing the program? What will you do if you have the temptation to cheat?*

What Do You Want
Your Life to Be Like?

I'm sure you don't want symptoms, but what do you want in life? The strongest emotion is stronger than any pain. We know this because soldiers injured in battle often don't need morphine or other strong pain relievers. Why is this? The happiness from being relieved from battle is more powerful than any discomfort.

You may have battled digestive symptoms for long periods of time. You may have tried strong drugs, and they have not solved the problem. *What can be your emotional high? Where are you going? How will you get there?* It might be helpful for you to do the relaxation exercise later in this chapter to relax fully. Then put on your favorite music, and brainstorm with a pen and paper before filling in the following form. What resources do you have to help you with these goals? What obstacles do you have in your way? How can you go over, around, through these obstacles?

Goals Worksheet			
	3 months	*1 year*	*3 years*
Family			
Career			
Physical			
Emotional			
Financial			
Spiritual			

Ask Yourself Better Questions

Many people with chronic health conditions ask themselves dis-empowering questions like these: Why me? How come I'm not like John, who can eat anything? When will I have to go to the hospital next? Why has God forsaken me? Negative thoughts are like toxic chemicals, they create waste. Ask yourself the following empowering questions if you get discouraged and at the beginning and end of each day. This alone will have a significant impact on your health.

What am I happy about? What am I proud about? What am I most grateful for? How could I treat myself as a good friend? What would that look like? How would that make me feel?

How could I enjoy exercise and stress reduction every day? How could I create more fun and joy in my life?

227

Keep Tempting Food Out of Reach

During weeks three and four it is crucial that you keep all tempting food out of reach, to avoid snacking and giving in to your cravings. The best option is to keep tempting food out of the house completely. If this is not possible because of your spouse or children, at least keep the tempting food such as cookies, snacks, and other junk food out of the refrigerator or pantry. Perhaps your spouse can keep the prohibited foods in a hiding place, or, better yet, can take the kids out for tempting food while you do something you enjoy.

Can You Communicate with Your Digestive System?

Let's review your digestive goals. Why do you want better digestion? Try to see your health as a puzzle you are trying to solve. See yourself as someone with a health "challenge" rather than as the victim of a cursed disease. Everyone has challenges. If you know someone who doesn't, I'd like to meet that person. Part of living in balance is that there will be times when things are better and times when things are worse. Can you accept any unpleasant feelings or sensations? Is your gut trying to tell you something? What is it telling you? When are you least likely to have symptoms? Could you eat or live like this all the time? What can you change? What resources or support do you have?

Understand the sensations your body is producing. Symptoms are usually the body's best attempt to heal. For example, abdominal cramping may be a sign that your body needs a break from food. Diarrhea may be a signal that your body cannot tolerate something, either a food or stress. Constipation is usually associated with stagnation, possibly a failure to "live and let live."

Intestinal gas is related to not being able to process food, and is often made worse by failure to exercise or process emotions. Can you pick a metaphor? For instance, if your discomfort were a color or shape, what would it look like? What does it feel like in there?

Can you move that sensation outside your body? If you ignore the signals of discomfort, the symptoms become stronger and more frequent. In order for the four weeks to work for you, it is important that you use your senses. The body has its own wisdom. When you tune in to your feelings, sensations, and thoughts, it becomes easier to interpret what your body is telling you.

Before Beginning the Program

When planning for the program, pick a month when you are not going to be traveling or entertaining. Visit your health professional to ensure that there is no reason you can't start a gradual exercise program, including abdominal exercises such as crunches. Set a date to begin the program, and stick to it. Rehearse the benefits every day. Think of the time you will save if you can manage your digestive symptoms instead of them managing you! Think of the goals you might achieve! It's time to begin making the transition to a cooked food diet. This step alone has helped many people manage digestive symptoms. Reduce alcohol consumption and substitute tea for coffee. Do you eat dairy products? Dairy products (milk, cream, cheese, yogurt, butter, and ice cream) are the number one digestive enemy. Have a sweet tooth? Until the program is formally under way, try to substitute fresh fruits for sweets such as candy, cookies, pastries, cake, chocolates, and so on.

You should use foods in the most natural state possible. As a general rule, if you can't pronounce the name of an ingredient, don't eat it. Food additives, yeast-containing foods such as mushrooms, wine, beer, bread, and nuts are problematic for many children and adults. Naturally occurring chemicals such as salicylates, the active ingredient in aspirin, and amines are poorly tolerated by many people (see this chapter). Although other tests are available that claim to evaluate sensitivities, they are expensive and do not have a long history of proven results. The rotation diet is the simplest, least expensive, and most reliable at determining sensitivity *for your body.*

Stress Reduction and Exercise

Stress reduction and exercise are an important part of healthy digestion. In today's busy world, many of us live in a "flight or fight" response. This is an arousal response and is the body's natural adaptation to stress; it's the body's best attempt to defend itself against a perception of some kind of danger. During stress, the body experiences heightened physiological, biochemical, and neurochemical responses, similar to the responses you would have if you were being chased by a tiger. Increased heart rate and blood pressure, muscle tension, and increased circulation to joints and muscles prepare the body to fight or run away. The body perceives stress as a danger signal and responds accordingly. Under daily stress, the gastrointestinal functions become compromised—you can't run from a tiger and digest food at the same time. Stress hormones are produced during stress and anxiety and act to prepare the body cells for increased activity. Stress hormones shut down digestive processes.

Incorporating a stress-reduction program and exercise into your daily routine will help you adapt to stress so that small annoyances do not result in excess upset, so that you "don't sweat the small stuff."

As mentioned earlier, before starting an exercise program, it's a good idea to visit a health professional to assess your baseline health and to find out if any exercises are contraindicated. Set aside twenty minutes or more each day for doing an enjoyable activity, vigorous enough that you are not dwelling on any problems. Walking is one of the best ways to begin an exercise program. Almost everyone can walk twenty minutes a day; no special place or equipment is required. Gardening also provides light exercise and is excellent for stress reduction. If you are in good shape, consider a vigorous activity such as swimming, a team sport, or an exercise class. In our clinic, we rarely see very athletic clients with digestive disorders, but if this is you, consider reducing your activity 50 percent or more. You might be exercising too much for your constitution.

Paul was a long-distance runner who had a diagnosis of ulcerative colitis. In addition to having many injuries that were slow to heal, he would have bouts of abdominal pain, diarrhea, and dehydration, which often resulted in hospitalization. Our advice to him was to reduce his rigorous training schedule and build up his body using herbs. In addition, he found the Digestive Clearing Program very useful as he learned that his body did not tolerate corn or wheat. Although Paul continues to run, he cross-trains more. Limiting the amount of wheat and corn he eats helps him to remain symptom free.

For stress reduction, we recommend meditation, prayer, yoga, or tai chi. The stress-reduction activity should be enjoyable to you. It's important that your spirit is in it; otherwise, it may not be beneficial. During the four-week program, we will present specific exercises that are stress reducing and beneficial for your digestive system. I have not met anyone who did not notice improvement after faithfully performing these exercises for thirty days. During the four weeks we will introduce you to two meditation techniques and abdominal self-massage.

Other Aspects of Food Sensitivities

Many patients have a difficult time digesting foods such as dairy products, beans, wheat, sweets, alcohol, and corn. The more you eat these foods, the more you are likely to become sensitive, as these products may cause a subclinical allergy, which degrades the intestinal lining over time. Even where the food is grown can affect your digestion. For example, many highly sensitive patients do better with locally grown organic foods than with commercially harvested products. Cooking also reduces sensitivities. It makes components in food easier to assimilate.

Several natural methods can be used to reduce food intolerance. Rotate your foods so that your diet has a lot of diversity. We have found certain supplements very useful. Taking an antioxidant containing mixed carotenes, vitamin C, vitamin E, zinc, and selenium may reduce your intolerance over time by improving the function of your immune system. Quercetin, enzymes, colostrum, and constitutional herbal therapy recommended by an herbalist can be extremely helpful. Quercetin has anti-allergic properties. Colostrum has immune factors that may make the body less allergic. Constitutional herbal therapy is used to make the body more resilient so that it can handle stress and food components more easily.

Changes in weather, particularly in the spring and fall, may trigger sensitivities. For example, you may tolerate eggs in the summer, but not in the winter, when the heater stirs up house dust. Barometric changes may also compromise health.

Environmental factors, such as where you work and live, may contribute to food intolerance. For example, moldy, windy, and damp environments may contribute to ill health and make the body more sensitive. Some patients have simultaneous allergy and sensitivity. Kirsten, for instance, had severe allergies to ragweed, herbs, and foods in the same family as ragweed. She also had sensitivities to dairy products, pork, and beans.

Cross-reactions are also possible — you may tolerate certain foods when they are eaten separately, but when combined, a reaction may result. I once saw a movie where the leading character had allergic symptoms when he drank tea and was exposed to cat dander. Needless to say, it took a long time to discover his cross-allergy. Your body may be sensitive to a combination of foods and another allergic substance such as pollen, house dust, mites, or mold. Other suspects include fuel oil, pets, particleboard, feather pillows, and chemicals or fumes.

Amines are naturally occurring nitrogen compounds in cheese, tomatoes, bananas, pineapples, and meat. Amines cause edema in the cranial area. Tyramine foods may be especially problematic: Aged strong cheese, chicken liver, pickled herring, and fava beans can cause such severe allergy that even smelling them can cause symptoms.

Getting Started

Choose to start the program during a month that works for you. Doing so will improve your chances of completing the program. Recall something that was difficult for you in the past that you completed — this will help you remember feelings of confidence. For many people, holidays and vacations are poor times to be on the Digestive Clearing Program.

There are two parts to the program. The first part involves changing your diet for the next thirty days; the second part involves lifestyle changes. The lifestyle changes should take no more than one hour per day. Many people have a hard time imagining spending another hour each day doing something. It is important, however, to understand that you are doing this to improve your digestive system—for life.

Some people wake up an hour earlier every day to gain that hour per day for stress reduction and exercise. You might find an extra hour by taking a monthlong break from the TV and news. You may even gain more than one hour a day! Listening to the news or watching TV does not necessarily improve your life.

The only thing you stand to lose is your digestive disorder.

Week One

For the next thirty days, the food you eat and drink should be warm or at room temperature. Avoid iced drinks and foods. Remove all cookies, crackers, margarine, vegetable shortening, prepared meats and fish (that is frozen or canned), shellfish, bread, corn, fruit juice, sodas, alcohol, and processed foods from the kitchen and house. Your diet should be free of wheat and dairy products. Three oils are allowed: extra virgin olive oil, sesame oil, and flaxseed oil if you have constipation. Eat more lean meats and freshwater fish. Substitute herbal teas and water for all other beverages. Drink at least 64 ounces of hot or room temperature water or herbal tea per day. Substitute fresh fruit for prepared sweets. If you drink coffee, start reducing your intake by half a cup per day until you are at one cup per day. For the duration of the program, no milk or cream is allowed in your coffee or tea. You may use the natural sweetener Stevia if you wish. Stevia can be found in most health food stores. Shop at a health food store to buy rice, millet, and other foods you may not normally eat. I recommend purchasing the herbal formula Quiet Digestion to help you digest and assimilate foods. Try to eat more vegetables, and drink herbal teas such as peppermint and chamomile. Drink ginger or cinnamon tea if you often feel cold or chilled. If you are currently taking medication, it is important that you not stop taking it without consulting your health professional. We also suggest you take probiotic supplements on an empty stomach twice per day. I recommend clients take them before bed and again in midmorning or midafternoon. Probiotics aid digestion and promote the absorption of nutrients. Acidophilus and bifidus are examples of popular probiotics. Recommended brands are PB-8, Natren, and Culturelle.

Begin the program today, and start walking. If you are on an exercise program, add walking to your regular routine on days you are not working out. Climb stairs instead of using elevators, and park your car farther from your destination and walk. Make a list of people you would enjoy exercising with. Could you exercise with your family?

Choose an activity that doesn't involve eating: for instance, movies, massage, a visit to the museum, or gardening. Purchase a journal or notebook and begin recording your meals, thoughts, and emotions. Spend twenty minutes daily doing the abdominal massage and twenty minutes or more exercising each day. If you have been exercising more than two hours a day, reduce your exercise level by half. It is important that while you are exercising you not think about your digestive system or any other problems.

- Spend twenty minutes a day doing abdominal massage. This is best accomplished in the morning or during a break in the daytime. Make sure you haven't eaten for at least two hours before doing the massage. See illustrations in Chapter Four for help doing the massage. If you wish, you can add a few drops of calming lavender essential oil to your abdomen during the massage. If you like, you can experiment with other essential oils such as peppermint; however, these should be diluted in olive oil. Use five drops of essential oil to one tablespoon of oil.

Week Two

By week two, you should have cut down to one cup of coffee or less per day. Limit your consumption of fruits and vegetables that are "not allowed" (in this chapter) as these tend to be gas producing. How are you dealing with stress? Start meditating or praying every day for twenty minutes in addition to your twenty-minute abdominal massage. If you have problems quieting your mind, I recommend yoga, tai chi, or audiovisual stimulators (www.mindmachines. com; 818-831-7931) to help you relax. It is important that if you pray, you pray for what you want. For example, say *Please help me to strengthen my body and improve my digestion.* This is also a good opportunity to give thanks for all the good things in your life.

Quiet your mind. Lie on the floor or sit up with your spine straight. With your in-breath, say *breathe deeply,* and with the out-breath say *relax completely.* To ensure that you are performing abdominal breathing correctly, place a book or hand on your abdomen. You should see a definite rise of your abdomen on the in-breath and lowering of your abdomen on the out-breath. An alternate stress-reduction exercise is the four-by-four breath. Breathe in for a count of four. Hold your breath for a count of four, then let your breath out for a count of four. Continue breathing in this fashion for twenty minutes. A more advanced version is to breathe in for a count of four, hold for four, breathe out for four, and hold your breath with your lungs empty for a count of four before breathing in.

Week Three and Four (Digestive Clearing Program)

It's now time to start the digestive clearing phase. Make sure that you are taking plenty of baths and probiotics. During weeks three and four, we urge you to discontinue any supplements (not mentioned in this book) that you are taking. The clearing plan is intended for those who have sensitivities. If you have severe reactions to any food, you should not consume that food even if it is on the list of acceptable foods. The following lists describe foods that are allowed and not allowed during weeks three and four.

Protein

Allowed: Beef, lamb, venison, elk, chicken, hen, turkey, duck, goose, ostrich, rabbit, pheasant, quail, and other game. Fresh fish.

Not allowed: Shellfish, prepared fish (such as breaded fish or fish sticks); prepared or preserved meats such as bacon, sausages, hotdogs, cold cuts, canned meats, pork, ham, and chicken eggs.

Preparation: Boiled, baked, broiled, and poached. Avoid deep-frying.

Vegetables

Allowed: Most. Limit potatoes to one per day.

Not allowed: Soybeans, tomatoes, cabbage, broccoli, cauliflower, mushrooms, brussels sprouts, beans, peas, lentils, and corn. These should be the first foods to be reintroduced.

Preparation: Try to use only fresh vegetables. Frozen vegetables may be used in a pinch. All vegetables should be steamed, boiled, or lightly stir-fried with olive oil. To do this, spray olive oil or use a maximum of one tablespoon per serving of extra virgin olive oil. Sesame and flax oils are also allowed; however, flax oil should not be heated.

Fruits

You may use lemon or lime wedges squeezed into hot or room temperature water. No other fruits are allowed. During the reintroduction phase (weeks five and after) begin with bananas, pears, apples, kiwi fruit, mangoes, papaya, pomegranates, passion fruit, guava, and melons. Blueberries, strawberries, raspberries, and other fruit may be added later.

Starches and Grains

Allowed: Rice, millet, amaranth, tapioca, buckwheat, and quinoa.

Not allowed: Wheat or wheat products, bread.

During the reintroduction phase add gluten-containing foods (oats, barley, rye, and spelt) and yeast-free muffins and crackers before adding breads.

Nuts

Eliminate nuts during the digestive clearing phase. During the reintroduction phase, you can start incorporating nuts and nut butters; however, peanuts and peanut butter should be tested last. Technically peanuts are in the bean (legume) family.

Seasoning, Flavorings, and Oils

Allowed: Sea salt, pepper, herbs, and spices, if they are used alone (that is, don't use combination seasonings). Use cold pressed extra virgin olive oil and sesame oil for cooking. Flax oil can be used unheated.

Not allowed: Red pepper, garlic, combination spices, artificial seasonings (if you can't pronounce it, don't eat it). Any oils besides olive, sesame, and flax.

Beverages

Allowed: Filtered water, spring water, carbonated water, and herbal tea. One cup a day of black or green tea may be used during weeks three and four, if necessary.

Prohibited Foods and Beverages

Not allowed: Any food not in the preceding lists, including but not limited to dairy products (milk, cream, butter, cheese, yogurt, ice cream), eggs, coffee, sweets, yeast, pastry, prepared or instant foods, vinegar, marmite (yeast extract), alcoholic beverages, canned foods, horseradish, bouillon, bread, wheat, corn, bagels, rolls, chips, salad dressing, desserts, fruits and fruit juices, iced drinks, iced foods, soda, uncooked foods, and green drinks such as barley green, spirilina, and algae.

The following are lists of additional foods and beverages to avoid.

Hidden Sources of Sugar

Some surprising sources of hidden sugar are:

bouillon	roasted nuts	peanut butter
canned and frozen foods	gravy	chips
tomato sauce	instant tea and coffee	salad dressings
	luncheon meats	soups

Here are some other names for sugar:

amasake
barley malt
beet sugar
brown rice syrup
brown sugar
cane juice
cane sugar
caramel color
carbitol
corn syrup
date sugar
dextrin
dextrose diglycerides
disaccharides
fructose
fruit juice sweetener
glucose
glycerin
glycerol
high-fructose
   corn syrup
honey
malt dextrin

malt extract
malt syrup
maltodextrin
maltodextrose
mannitol
mannose
maple syrup
molasses
monoglycerides
monosaccharides
powdered sugar
raisins (sweetened)
raw sugar
rice malt
rice syrup
sorbitol
succanat
sucrose
sugar cane
turbinado
xylitol
zylose

⁂ Sweets ⁂

Cake
Candy
Cereal
Cookies
Doughnuts
French toast
Graham crackers

Ice cream
Jams
Pastries
Pies
Preserves
Waffles

✻ Wheat Products ✻

Beer
Biscuits
Bouillon
Bread
Bulgur
Cereal
Chips
Crackers
Croutons
Couscous
Dumplings
Durum
Farina
Flour (white and whole wheat)
French toast
Fried foods
   (coating/batter)
Gin
Luncheon meats
Malt

MSG
Muffins
Noodles
Ovaltine
Pancake mix
Pasta
Pizza
Popovers
Postum
Pretzels
Rolls
Sauces
Sausage
Semolina
Soy sauce, tamari
Stuffing
Waffles
Wheat germ
Whiskey

✻ Yeast Products ✻

Antibiotics derived from yeast
   (Chloromycetin, mycin
   drugs, penicillin,
   tetracycline)
Barbecue sauce
Biscuits
Bread crumbs
Brewer's yeast
Buns
B vitamins (yeast)

Catsup
Cheese
Citric acid
Crackers
Dried fruits
Dry roasted nuts
Fermented beverages: beer,
   brandy, gin, rum, whiskey,
   wine, vodka
Grapes

Yeast, continued

Malted products: candy, cereals, malted milk
Moldy melon
MSG
Mushrooms
Mustard
Pizza
Prepared cheese products
Salad dressings
Pretzels
Sour cream
Soy sauce
Stuffing
Torula (a type of yeast)
Vinegar
Vitamins made from yeast
Yeast extract (bouillon)

✣ Corn Products ✣

Baby foods
Beer, ale, brandy, wine
Candy (corn-sweetened)
Carbonated beverages
Cereal
Corn chips
Cornmeal
Corn oil
Cornstarch
Corn sugar (dextrose)
Corn syrup (glucose)
Frostings
Fructose
Fruit juices
Fruits (canned, frozen)
Gelatin
Glucose
Gravy
Grits
Gum
Ham
High-fructose corn syrup
Hominy
Ice cream
Jam, preserves
Jello
Lozenges
Maize
Margarine
MSG
Nescafe
Pancake syrup
Peanut butter (corn-sweetened)
Polenta
Popcorn
Powdered sugar
Preservatives
Processed luncheon meats and sausages

Corn Products, *continued*

Pudding
Saccharin
Salad dressings
Sandwich spreads
Salt (iodized)
Sauces
Seasonings
Sherbets
Soda

Sorbitol
Soup
Soy milk
Tortillas
Vegetables (canned, frozen)
Vinegar
Xanthan gum
Yogurt

❊ Soy Products ❊

Artificial meat (gluten or soy)
Bean sprouts
Lecithin
Margarine
Meat substitute fast food
Miso
Protein powder
Salad dressings
Soybean flour
Soybean oil

Soybeans
Soy pasta
Soy sauce
Soy sprouts
Soy vegetable oil and broth
Tempeh
Tofu
Tuna or other fish packed in
    oil
Vegetable protein

❊ Egg Products ❊

Custards
Deviled eggs
Doughnuts
Dried eggs
Egg albumin (ovalbumin)
Egg Beaters
Eggnog
Egg whites

Egg yolks
French toast
Frostings
Fruit pie
Mayonnaise
Muffins
Omelets
Pancakes

Egg products, continued

Pasta	Quiche
Pastry	Soufflés
Powdered eggs	Tartar sauce
Puddings	

❧ Milk Products ❧

Au gratin potatoes	Lactose
Buttermilk	Powdered milk
Carob products	Pudding
Casein	Salad dressing
Cheese	Sherbet
Chocolate	Skim milk
Cream	Sodium caseinate
Ice cream	Sour cream
Kefir	Whey
Lactalbumin	Whipped cream
Lactate	Yogurt
Lactoglobulin	

Reintroduction Phase:
Weeks Five and Thereafter

We recommended that you stay on the clearing plan and proceed in the suggested order. Keep a journal and record food, liquids, supplements, moods, and symptoms. Use colored pens to highlight adverse reactions so that they stand out, and use a numbering system: 0 (no reaction) to 10 (can't tolerate). Reintroduce foods that you know or feel will be the most tolerable first. When reintroducing foods, make sure to get one or two healthy servings. If you react to a food, avoid it and reintroduce it again in two to three weeks. If a food produces a minor reaction, avoid it for three months; if a major reaction occurs, avoid the food for six months and then reintroduce it. A mild reaction may be indigestion, gas, bloating, loose stools or discomfort. A major reaction may be watery or explosive diarrhea, difficulty moving your bowels (prolonged constipation), constant gas, or pain. You may have problems with a food family, or your problem may be specific to a type of food. For instance, Yukon gold potatoes may create problems, but not red potatoes; one type of apple may produce a reaction, but not other types. The problem could be related to pesticides or the way the food is cooked; for instance, cooked carrots may not create a problem, but raw carrots may cause gas.

Below is a suggested reintroduction order. Items at the top of the list should be tested first. Foods at the bottom of the list should be tested last.

In the following list, you should have no more than one serving per day of items marked with an asterisk (*) and no more than one serving every three days of items marked with a double asterisk (**).

- Prohibited vegetables (unless you know they are problematic), except tomatoes and tomato products; not beans or legumes. These should be tested later.
- Whole fruits (except berries, melon, grapes, and dried fruits). Fruits should always be consumed on an empty stomach, not with meals, for digestive health.
- Eggs.*
- Vinegar and mustard. If you cannot tolerate vinegar, try buffered vitamin C in powdered form as a substitute.
- Oats, barley, rye, spelt, triticale, teff, kamut (gluten-containing grains). Many people who can't tolerate wheat can tolerate these grains. Try eating them in cooked form.
- Nonwheat pasta.*
- Butter* (for recipes). Occasionally butter may be used as a flavoring agent, but we want to avoid using butter with

everything (for example, butter with toast, as an ingredient in a rich dessert, in meat or vegetable sauce, and so on).

- Beans, including soy products.* (You may find it easier to digest miso and tempeh rather than tofu, soybeans, soy milk.)
- Mushrooms (test all mushrooms before button mushrooms—they are most likely to get mold).
- Yeast-free and wheat-free muffins, yeast-free and wheat-free crackers.
- Pork and ham.
- Melon, berries, grapes. Make sure there is no white fungus. These fruits are to be tested later because they easily get fungal mold.
- Corn and corn products.* (Test fresh corn first.)
- Goat and sheep cheese.** (Occasionally goat and sheep's milk can be added to recipes, but they are not recommended with cereal or as beverages.)
- Raw vegetables.* (Be sure to chew well. Some people can only tolerate salads and other raw vegetables in the summer months.)
- Other fresh foods not mentioned in this list.

Tips: If you find that you are having increased symptoms since starting weeks three and four of the program, you may need to consult the food family lists in Appendix B. It may be helpful to test in order of food families before going to the next family; of course, it's smart to test families of food that you like. You do not need to test foods that you never eat or are unlikely to eat.

You should consume the following foods every three days or less if you are having digestive symptoms:

- Cereal. Cold cereal with milk is one of the most difficult things to digest. Try oatmeal porridge and other hot grain porridges instead of cold cereal with milk. By adding more water, you can thin the porridge so that milk is not needed.

- Peanuts, nuts, and nut butters. (These can be highly allergic for some people. Their high fat content makes them difficult to digest.)
- Cheese from cow's milk.
- Shellfish.
- Wheat (breads, bulgur, couscous), wheat pasta.
- Sweets and sweeteners (for example, honey, pure maple syrup, date extract, molasses, sorghum). It's always better to increase protein-rich foods or protein shakes or eat tolerable whole fruits to counter sweet cravings. You may find eating yams or taking chromium supplements (200 to 600 mcg per day) useful. L-Glutamine (500-3000 mg) may also be useful to counter food cravings. Some people will notice an immediate benefit, others will notice results over time. Tonic herbs recommended by an herbalist can also help.
- Diluted fruit juice. Undiluted fruit juices should not be consumed.
- Sodas.
- Tomatoes and tomato products. (Some people will do better with fresh tomatoes in season than commercial products such as tomato sauces.)
- Luncheon meats, sausage, and bacon.
- Prepared foods; frozen, canned, deli, or restaurant foods.
- Alcoholic beverages. (If you must drink, you might find that some types are easier on your system than others, as different grains, processing, and preservatives are used.)
- Commercial spices with multiple ingredients.
- For health reasons we only recommend extra virgin olive oil, sesame oil, and flax oil. If you are intolerant of these ingredients, consider other oils.

Not recommended: green foods (algae, spirulina), raw vegetables in the winter and cooler months, cow's milk, ice cream, pizza, fast food, eating in restaurants or delis habitually, and MSG and other additives.

Digestion-Clearing Meal Plan

You may notice that the meal plan includes some familiar as well as some unusual foods. It is highly important that you eat a varied diet and rotate the foods you do eat. I tried to include selections from meat, poultry, and fish. You may want to include venison and rabbit, as they fulfill the requirements for lean sources of protein. The rare foods list in Appendix B includes other more exotic meats. When selecting breakfast and lunch choices, it is important that you rotate the grains you eat. Many digestive patients seem to do well on cooked grain breakfasts; however, whenever possible you should not eat the same grain at every meal. We always want to keep rotation in mind. Therefore, if you eat one grain on one day, the following day or meal, you would consume a different grain. The meal plan described later is meant to be a guide. If you don't like a food mentioned or your body does not tolerate it, there is no need to incorporate it. The criteria for all meals should be that they are low in fat, moderate in lean protein, with plenty of digestible vegetables and alternate grains that do not contain gluten.

Coping Strategies

You may find after reading this book that going to the supermarket is a frustrating experience, as it seems like everything contains wheat, corn, or milk. Many of us also may associate these foods with good things such as mothers, farms, wholesomeness, or even the American way of life. Never fear, however; there are many exciting substitutes. When you are finished with the preparation, clearing phase, and reintroduction phase of the program, you will have a better insight as to which foods your body does and does not tolerate. Coupled with stress-reduction and exercise, you have an excellent chance of going from a person whose digestive system controls you, to a person who controls your digestive system. You may find after several months that you don't need be so strict with yourself, as long as you eat a healthy variety of foods. Occasionally "blowing it" will not be a problem, especially if you take Digestive Harmony herbal supplement before and after the offending food. Using the recommended probiotic products will help rebuild your digestive system. Over time we hope you will realize that it is possible to eat around the aisles of the supermarket where the fresh foods are. Hopefully you will have found coping strategies around family, friends, and coworkers.

It is important not to dwell on the things you won't be eating, but rather to make this an experience of trying new things. During the clearing phase, we introduce alternative grains such as rice, millet, buckwheat, and quinoa. There are recipes for rabbit and lamb. Are there vegetables you have forgotten about and could be enjoying?

Some people will want to prepare several dinners at once, which saves quite a bit of time, and bring extra portions to work, where the food can be reheated. Most of the recipes in this book freeze well. Other people will want even greater variety, so meal plans also include lunch and breakfast ideas. The foundation of the program is soups, stews, and porridges. I firmly believe that if your digestion isn't working, the only way to change it is to take different actions. Why not try eating your heaviest meal of the day for breakfast or lunch, and your lightest at dinner? In other words, as the old adage says, "eat like a prince for breakfast, a merchant for lunch, and a pauper for dinner." What else could you change? Is there a friend, family member, or colleague who would want to do the program with you? Many people find that they can lose or maintain healthy weight on the diet, and people with chronic fatigue or chronic muscle pain (fibromyalgia syndrome) have also noticed better digestion, increased energy, and less pain.

Meal Plans

In the following food list, an asterisk indicates items of which you should not have more than one serving per day:

Breakfast Ideas

Chicken or beef soup
Buckwheat (soba) noodles
Yam
Rice or millet porridge
Baked potatoes*
Quinoa

Lunch/Snack

Anchovies, mackerel, tuna, sardines (packed in water only)
Beef, lamb, or turkey burger
Yam or sweet potato
Rice cakes
Buckwheat (soba)
Chicken, beef, or vegetable soup
Steamed or stir-fried vegetables or vegetable puree
Baked potatoes*

Slice of home-cooked chicken or turkey
Artichoke

Beverages

Water with mint, cucumber, or slice of lemon or lime
Herbal tea, especially ginger or cinnamon (use if you often feel cold or chilled), peppermint, chamomile, or green or black tea (one cup per day)
Carbonated water (natural flavoring okay)

Dinner

Steak, quinoa, and zucchini casserole
Turkey breast, squash, and wild rice
Halibut, sweet potatoes, and vegetable soup
Stir-fried turkey with vegetables, yams, and artichokes
Pot roast, potatoes, and carrots
Lamb roast, wild rice and herbs, butternut squash
Cod, rice, and greens
Chicken breasts, quinoa, and roasted vegetables
Salmon, wild rice, and vegetable soup
Beef with buckwheat (soba) noodles and beets
Rabbit, potatoes, and carrots
Lamb chops, millet, and vegetable soup
Veal medallions, vegetable puree
Roast turkey, rice, and beets

Appendix A

Commonly Asked
Questions and Answers

This appendix includes questions with answers submitted by readers and practitioners after the first edition.

Diet

- *What about reducing carbohydrates for people with digestive disorders?*

Low carbohydrate diets are currently very popular for people who are overweight or have diabetes and pre diabetes known as syndrome X. Although they have not been widely studied for people with digestive disorders in the U.S., in developing countries where people use less refined carbohydrates (i.e., packaged foods), there is much less incidence of digestive disorders, especially colon disorders. On the other hand, vegetables are very healthy foods, and sometimes we find clients at our clinic who go on the "Atkins type" diets, do not eat enough vegetables, and may go overboard on fats such as dairy products like cream and cheese. These are clearly not healthy foods for people with digestive disorders, and scare people from eating relatively healthy foods such as carrots because they are high on the glycemic index. What is missing is balance. In my experience, the best diet for people with digestive disorders is plenty of vegetables, lean protein, and I suggest experimenting with alternative grains and fruits. For more information, please see the Digestive Clearing Plan chapter.

- *I seem to be supersensitive. Some food allergy books even suggest rotating cooking oils. Do you recommend this?*

Supersensitive people may benefit from rotating cooking oils. This book focuses on the special needs of people with digestive disorders. My research has led to the conclusion that olive oil is the best all-around oil for most people for cooking and dressings. Sesame oil and flax oil are also good.

- *I'm allergic to beef and pork. What should I do?*

You might try to get hormone-free variations of these meats and see if you notice any difference. Rather than just eating white meat and fish, to get a side spectrum of nutrients try various protein sources listed as rare foods in Appendix B.

- *I'm a vegetarian. What can I do?*

I would urge you to look at the reasons why you are a vegetarian. Vegetarianism is great for people who live in hot climates and who do not do much physical or mental work; otherwise it may be difficult. It is always good to rotate one's diet, and most of us need to eat more vegetables. Vegetarians in the West often rely too much on dairy products, grains, and beans. The only way you can follow the digestive clearing program is by trying to find rice protein without additives, otherwise it is simply not possible to get adequate protein, as beans are out. You may find that your body is able to tolerate meat better than you think, particularly if you stick to soups and stews and fish. Many of our clients who switch from a vegetarian diet to the Digestive Clearing Program with fish and meat in the form of soups and stews a few days a week do quite well. Other options would be to see an herbalist so that you can take herbs to give you ample energy, or to take amino acid supplements that contain all the basic amino acids. Note that amino acids should be taken under professional supervision. If you have been a vegetarian for a long period, I suggest that you get tested for anemia and Vitamin B_{12} deficiency.

- *Have you heard about food sensitivity tests?*

Although food allergies can be diagnosed, the best way to diagnose food sensitivities is by the rotation diet. For more information, see the Digestive Clearing Plan in this book. There are tests that claim to reveal your food sensitivities. At best they can serve as a starting point. In other words, if the tests show sensitivity to pork, you can eliminate pork from your diet and see if this makes a difference in your digestive health. In our clinic, we have found these tests to be expensive and unreliable.

- *Will I ever be able to eat wheat and dairy products?*

After a period of avoiding these foods, it may be possible to eat these foods every three days or so, particularly if you are rebuilding the gastrointestinal system with herbs and probiotics. The chief problem we see with clients is they put these foods into their diets much too quickly, and this may trigger a return of symptoms. If eliminating these foods has brought an absence of discomfort, try to eat them once every three days or less.

- *I have a friend who said that when she got a water filter, her digestive symptoms stopped.*

We always recommend our clients drink filtered water, as tap water can contain unsafe bacteria, heavy metals, and parasites. I have heard it reported that sulfites in the water supply can cause digestive symptoms. The best and most expensive form of water filtration is called reverse osmosis. These systems must be installed by a professional. Camping stores often have portable water filters, which can be used in the home as well.

- *My doctor says I'm not lactose intolerant, but every time I drink milk or eat ice cream I experience cramping or diarrhea. If I do stop eating dairy foods, how do I maintain adequate calcium intake?*

Although you may not be intolerant to lactose, you may be intolerant to one or more of the other constituents in milk. Therefore, it may be prudent to stop all dairy products. To assure adequate calcium intake, consider taking a calcium supplement, preferably in absorbable form such as citrate or aspartate. If you want to use magnesium to aid in the absorption of calcium, take half as much magnesium as calcium; if you suffer from stress, hypertension, or constipation, take equal amounts of calcium and magnesium. Start out at a reduced dosage and slowly increase. If you have problems with one brand or form of calcium, try another. There are additional cofactors, which may help bone density; they are zinc, copper, manganese, vitamin K, boron, and folic acid. Foods rich in calcium include soy products (if you can tolerate them), turnip greens, kale, black-eyed peas, sesame seeds, okra, bok choy, figs, dried apricots, almonds, broccoli, and amaranth.

- *What do you mean by dairy products?*

Milk, cream, cheese, butter, and ice cream. Yogurt is also a dairy product, however homemade yogurt or brands which have acidophilus and probiotics ("live cultures") are frequently the most easily tolerated.

- *What are the drawbacks of bread?*

Many breads contain wheat, which is a common allergen, and yeast, which many people are sensitive to. Bread is also often associated with unhealthy foods. For example, butter, mayonnaise, and margarine are usually spread on bread. The first two contain excessive fat, and margarine contains trans-fatty acids, which should not be consumed at all. Additionally, bread is ordinarily used to make sandwiches that contain foods like cheese and luncheon meat, which are high in fat, salt, preservatives, and additives. To avoid these unhealthy foods, substitute crackers or muffins that are wheat-free for bread, and instead of luncheon meat, use meat that you cooked from scratch. This is much healthier, delicious, and easier to digest than cheese and luncheon meat.

- *Does this mean that I can't go out for a drink with my friends?*

During the four weeks, alcohol is prohibited. You might want to make other suggestions while you are on the program. As long as you are careful to bring food ahead of time, there are hundreds of activities you can share with friends.

- *I tried the anti-candida diet once, and it didn't work that well. Why not?*

The anti-candida diet works for many people. For others, it is not balanced enough. Some of the products that are recommended with the anti-candida diet (for example, caprylic acid) are hard on the digestive system. Finally, many people have problems with candida because their digestive systems are weak. Our program is designed to strengthen the digestive system. Constitutional herbal therapy is also very helpful, but you need to see an herbalist to pursue this route.

- *I often travel for work. Can I do the program while traveling?*

The two-week clearing phase needs to be done at home. While theoretically the first two weeks and the reintroduction could be done while traveling, it's very difficult to do so. Sometimes you have to choose between health and a career. I suggest that you make every effort to at least pick a three-week period when you can do the program at home. This would be the two-week clearing phase and a week of rotating foods. If you truly get stuck, go to a restaurant and have meat, poultry, or fish with nothing added. Baked and boiled potatoes or steamed vegetables are usually safe.

- *Does it take a long time to cook all these foods?*

It may take longer than going to delis. However, not only will your gut thank you, your heart will thank you also. There are strategies that help make cooking less time-consuming. For example, you can cook the majority of the week's food on Sunday, or at the same time that you roast vegetables you can bake a roast and cook soup. Like many parts of the program, it's essential that you keep remembering the benefits, not the difficulties, if you want to succeed in healing your digestive system.

- *Will I be on this diet the rest of my life?*

No. It is meant to be a starting point. The goal is to find out which foods seem to be aggravating your digestive system. Hopefully you will be learning about new foods that you can incorporate into your diet so that your diet is more varied. Also, in time you will learn which foods your body absolutely does not tolerate, and which foods can be incorporated every three days instead of every day.

- *I live in an area where there are no natural food stores. How can I get some of the foods that you mention?*

You can get many of the foods mentioned in this book via mail order. Some of my clients who live in rural areas need to stock up on some of the staples during trips to the city. They are lucky because they can grow much healthier produce than can be found in stores.

- *Will people make fun of the way I'm eating? Truck drivers can't eat rice cakes!*

First of all, you don't need to eat with other people, especially if they are going to be insulting. Announce to everybody that you are eating differently on "doctor's orders." Other people don't have to know that you are referring to your inner doctor.

- *I eat only chicken and fish, yet I see that your meal plan includes a lot of red meat. Why?*

Chicken and fish are good, but you may be missing nutrients only found in red meat and game. I am trying to emphasize the point of eating a more varied diet. It is also possible that by limiting your diet, you may develop sensitivities to chicken and fish.

- *What about cooking for my spouse?*

I suggest that you put all cookies, crackers, and so on on a shelf that you can't reach. I'm sure that your spouse would like most of the delicious and nutritious foods you will be serving.

- *Can I use soy milk?*

During the clearing phase (weeks 3 and 4) beans and bean products such as soy milk are excluded. While beneficial for many people, especially menopausal women, and less allergenic than milk, many people with digestive disorders are intolerant to beans. As it is highly concentrated, soy milk may present an additional problem. If you enjoy soy products, you may consider testing them earlier than is indicated during the reintroduction phase.

Herbs & Supplements

- *What is the best way to take probiotics? Can they be taken at the same time as antibiotics?*

Probiotics are best taken on an empty stomach. In addition,

it is a good idea to rotate probiotic products. This is to introduce a variety of healthy organisms to the digestive tract. In our clinic, we recommend at least two weeks of probiotics for every week of antibiotic use. We recommend probiotics to be taken while clients are on antibiotics; however, we recommend that they be taken at least two hours apart.

- *What is Saccharomyces boulardii?*

This is nutritional yeast that is usually used to stop diarrhea. In four weeks of treatment, a remission was seen in 68 percent of patients with ulcerative colitis who were maintained on Asacol (mesalamine) but were unsuitable candidates for steroid treatment. Subjects took 250 mg three times a day. Remissions were confirmed by endoscope (Suslandi M, Giollo P, Testonic PA. A pilot trial of Saccharomyces boulardii in ulcerative colitis. Eur J Gastroenterol hepatol. 2003: 15 (6): 697-8).

- *Are food enzymes addicting?*

There are two main types of digestive enzymes: animal and vegetable. Both types of enzymes can be useful in order to help food digest. Therefore, typically, enzymes are taken with a meal to prevent indigestion, intestinal gas, and bloating. Certain people may notice they have improved stools after taking digestive enzymes. What I have noticed is that after several months, the body seems to become dependent on enzymes, which then can make digesting food without them difficult. On the other hand, taken symptomatically they can be helpful when restaurants or unfamiliar food are unavoidable. Enzymes can also be used until more constitutional approaches take hold. For example, if one has cold signs, warming herbs can be taken between meals while enzymes are taken with food. Over a period of a few weeks or months, the enzymes are no longer necessary, as the herbs have corrected the constitutional imbalance.

- *What will it take to make herbs and supplements more acceptable to mainstream physicians?*

A frequent complaint is that the alternative and complementary approaches are not researched enough. What the skeptics are referring to is the lack of double blind placebo controlled studies where neither the doctor nor the patient knows who is getting the active substance and who is getting the sugar pill. One problem with this type of research is that it is very expensive. Oftentimes researchers only research what drug companies pay them to research; and so many of these researchers are biased against herbs and nutritional interventions, particularly since they don't pay the bills. Surgery and many other methods used by doctors are not always proven with double blind studies, however, doctors utilize these techniques because they believe that they are valuable. In contrast, they tend not to use alternative approaches because they don't believe they are effective. It must be realized that the historical usage of herbs may be of even greater importance, as often double blind studies fail to anticipate problems that show up as the medications are dispensed in real life.

One encouraging sign is that most medical schools in the U.S. have an elective course in alternative medicine. In time, patients will bring their stories to doctors and hopefully they will be more open to alternatives. Finally, the greatest area for alternative approaches is for prevention. If people use herbal medicines as a first approach instead of a last ditch effort, the success of alternative approaches will be unparalleled.

- *I'm reluctant to tell my doctor that I'm taking herbal remedies. What should I do?*

Surveys have found that one in three Americans uses some form of alternative therapy. It is important for you to explain to your doctor that herbal therapies are meant to be used along with conventional modalities, and that you hope he/she will support you. If not, then you might consider going to a different doctor.

- *Aren't Chinese herbs better for Chinese and Western herbs better for Westerners?*

Not necessarily. In the U.S. alone, millions have used traditional Chinese healing methods, including herbs and acupuncture, with satisfaction. Chinese herbology is more complex and difficult to learn; for practitioners to apply it successfully, they must learn an entire healing system. Therefore, it is not suitable for self-treatment. Western herbology, on the other hand, is not quite so involved, and can be used for self-treatment.

- *What do you do if the triple therapy for H. pylori doesn't work?*

Many clients who come to our clinic have tried the drug approach to treating ulcers and have found that it doesn't always work. For one thing, H. pylori is probably a very common bacteria that occurs in both people who have ulcers and people who do not have ulcer symptoms. Although bismuth preparations can play a role in healing the ulcers or alleviating some of the symptoms, antibiotics can lead to other complications, including fungal overgrowth, antibiotic resistance, and a reduction of healthy intestinal bacteria. Most likely triple therapy works for clients who are relatively healthy. In clients who have multiple health problems, antibiotic therapy for ulcers can make other conditions worse. In the case where triple therapy does not work, we often need to use good probiotic products, tonic herbs, and specific herbs like licorice, which heal the stomach and intestines. In most of these cases, we can help someone who has failed triple therapy.

- *Have you heard of mastic gum?*

Mastic gum (Pistacia lentiscus) is a European remedy used to heal ulcers, H. pylori, and heartburn. The general dosage is 1-2 grams per day.

- *How about taking vitamins?*

I usually recommend high-quality, hypoallergenic supplements. If you have been taking a product and still have digestive problems, it makes sense to stop what you are taking and then reintroduce a different supplement during the reintroduction phase.

IBS/IBD Questions

- *Are there any answers for pouchitis?*

About 1.5 million people in the U.S. have had their large intestines removed. A pouch can be created from the small intestine, so that it is possible to go to the bathroom normally, and a colostomy bag is avoided. The main problem with this procedure is the pouch can become inflamed. Other complications include gas and stool incontinence in about one third of the people who have this procedure. Approximately twenty percent need to have an additional surgery.

Pouchitis or inflammation of the ileal pouch is usually treated with antibiotics. In order to prevent inflammation from occurring, probiotics will help. In addition, probiotics will reduce intestinal gas.

- *I am a female with IBS who has frequent diarrhea. My physician suggested taking a prescription drug, Lotronex, however I was afraid of the side effects. Now I mostly just suffer, as I get headaches from the over-the-counter medication, Imodium.*

Colostrom can be experimented with. Starting dosage is generally 1 to 2 grams taken three or more times per day. Maintenance dosage is 1 to 2 grams per day. In addition, herbalists can recommend constitutional herbal formulas mentioned in the text, which can also treat your symptoms. As you suffer from diarrhea, it is very important that you drink plenty of water. You may also find the Digestive Clearing Diet helps you identify which foods may be contributing to the diarrhea.

- *Is there a role for antidepressants in the treatment of IBS?*

Although the newer SSRI antidepressants such as Prozac tend to irritate the gastrointestinal tract, the older medications called tricyclics have antispasmodic and pain-relieving effects. They are also sedating. Examples of tricyclic antidepressants include Elavil (amitriptyline) and Valium. They are considered highly addictive. Typical side effects include constipation, dry mouth, dizziness, tiredness, weight gain, and sexual dysfunction.

The best antidepressant is exercise. Exercising to one's own level of health is the single best way to improve one's digestion. If a client is already exercising and is able to avoid trigger foods such as dairy products and wheat, the next thing to try would be to use an herbal formula that has antispasmodic and analgesic effects. Such an approach may produce slower results than pharmaceutical antidepressants. However, there are fewer side effects. In addition, I have clients who have been able to be weaned off tricyclics using herbs. Typically they have gotten comparable clinical results, without the grogginess that can accompany the use of tricyclics.

- *My cousin, who has Crohn's disease, went to a medical clinic specializing in alternative medicine. She was administered antibiotics to kill the TB bacteria as well as a bag full of supplements. With the tests that doctor ordered, the cost was several thousand dollars. Although for a short time things seemed to help, after several weeks she seemed to have a flare-up. Once she stopped everything her health was restored. Care to comment?*

Some practitioners believe that Crohn's disease may be caused by a type of TB bacteria (Mycobacterium paratuberculosis) or bacteria that has not been identified yet. Therefore, antibiotics are administered. It is unclear whether it was the antibiotics or the "bag full of supplements" that seemed to cause a flare up. I have noticed that some alternative doctors practice "shotgun" pharmacy. The problem with this approach, administering everything that might be helpful for a condition, is the digestive system can be compromised with too much of a good thing. I prefer not to administer too many things at one time. Just because your cousin had one bad experience, rest assured this does not reflect on all alternative approaches. As in Western medicine, there are good practitioners and bad practitioners. Complementary approaches are very subjective. A good practitioner for one person or condition might not be appropriate for another patient.

- *If my client has his intestines partially or entirely removed, can herbal medicine still work?*
At our clinic, we have treated many people who have had all or parts of their intestines removed. In most cases we are able to help improve the symptoms of these clients. As gastrointestinal function is compromised, we usually select teas or tablets that are tested to break down quickly in the gastrointestinal tract.

- *I'm on TPN [total parenteral nutrition]. Can I still use herbs and other nutritional supplements?*
If you are able to drink fluids, you can use herbs in tea form, either by preparing traditional decoctions, or by grinding herbal tablets in a powder and infusing them in boiling water. Choose vitamin supplements in powder form as well, or for those that come in capsules, break open the capsules, and add to water or a nutritional powder. I strongly suggest working with a health professional who is experienced with herbs and supplements.

Miscellaneous Questions

- *I seem to get heartburn every time I swallow pills.*

Usually you can prevent digestive reactions by taking pills one at a time with plenty of water before taking the next pill. If you are taking tablets, it may be possible to divide the pills in two with a butcher knife before swallowing.

- *Colon cancer runs in my family. Is there anything I can do to prevent it?*

A person is twice as likely to get colon cancer if they have a parent or sibling with the disease. Data from the Nurses Health Study shows that a diet high in folic acid and methionine (an amino acid) and low in alcohol for five years showed reduced colon cancer risk. Women consuming at least 400 mcg per day of folic acid virtually eliminated their risk of inheritable colon cancer (Fuch CS et al. The influence of folate and multivitamin use on the familial risk of colon cancer in women. *Cancer Epidemiol Biomarkers Prev.* 2002: 11 (3): 227-34).

Folic acid also protects against heart disease and birth defects. It is typically found in green leafy vegetables and is also found in supplements. Methionine is found in meat and fish and is also found in the supplement SAMe (S-adenosyl-methionine).

Antioxidant vitamins may help reduce the recurrence of polyps. In seventy-two patients, those who took antioxidant vitamins showed a decrease in the recurrence of intestinal polyps as compared with a control group that did not receive the vitamins. Subjects received 30,000 IU of vitamin A, 1 gram of vitamin C, and 70 mg (approximately 100 IU) of vitamin E (*Letsliveonline.com,* March 2002).

Calcium in supplement form may also have a preventive effect on colon cancer. In an American Cancer Society study of 60,000 men and women taking between 700 to 1,200 mg per day of total calcium, had a decreased risk of colon cancer (*Cancer Causes and Control,* 2003: 14: 1–12). Ideally you would also eat as many vegetables and fruits as you can tolerate, as these have a cancer protective effect.

- *Which digestive conditions are more difficult to treat?*

Generally, congenital diseases, that is, conditions that run in families, prove harder to treat than acquired ones. The sooner you visit a holistic practitioner after your symptoms appear, the better the prognosis.

- *How should children's digestive conditions be addressed?*

Youngsters who can adopt dietary changes often make quick progress. The child and family must make the choice of whether or not to undertake dietary changes or to stay on medications. I was once consulted by a 10 year-old boy with Crohn's disease and his family. The biomedical solution was to have the boy take Prednisone and immune suppressives long-term. I indicated to the family that unless the boy eliminated his daily milk drinking and tomato products (the family was Italian), that he would probably have to remain on these medications.

Also, for such cases, I recommend ongoing counseling, either family therapy or spiritual counseling, to encouraging the child to participate in extracurricular activities and exercise.

- *Why does something that I tried in the past no longer work?*

Our bodies are constantly changing, as is our health. Our health is dependent on stages of illness, stress load, climate, and diet. Therefore, these changes can affect the efficacy of whatever therapy we are using. In addition to the fluctuations of our body and environment, our bodies become accustomed to medications and supplements, including herbs, that we take. This is why traditional herbalists frequently modify the herbal formula that a patient is taking. With the help of a practitioner, you can explore ways to change your life so that you can be symptom-free.

- *I was doing really well, then things stopped working. Now I'm discouraged. What should I do?*

First I would look at any recent changes. These could be ways in which your diet or stress load has changed. Weather changes and biorhythms (circadian rhythms) can contribute to changes in digestive health. Some clients notice that things can go downhill after several days of rain or if they are in indoor environments that are excessively cold or damp. You may need to try to get more exercise and take herbs such as ginger that help fight the cold and dampness. Digestive Harmony also helps. It is important to realize this is a temporary setback; things are not going downhill.

- *I got this book for a loved one. Unfortunately, that person seems more interested in telling me why this won't work than in trying the program. What can I do?*

This is very common. There is not a lot of support in our culture for people who have successfully treated themselves for chronic digestive disorders. The medical community shrugs and doesn't encourage these people to be more vocal. All most doctors know about are drugs and surgery. That is not the purpose of this book, which is promoting digestive health and encouraging changes.

If you need a more specialized book, I recommend *Allergy Cooking with Ease* by Nicolette Dumke and *The Whole Way to Allergy Relief and Prevention* by Jacqueline Krohn, MD

- *What if I am already underweight?*

If you are underweight, it is very important that you eat adequate protein. You may consider meat soups in the morning if possible during the clearing phase. If you can get pure rice protein without added sweeteners, this would make an easy-to-digest breakfast. After the two-week clearing phase, you might want to test soy earlier than most people, as soy can be a good source of vegetable protein. Traditionally, corn is used to help people gain weight, so this may be another food you could consider testing earlier than most people. However, keep in mind that many people with digestive symptoms react to both soy and corn.

- *I did exactly what was recommended, but I still have symptoms. What is wrong?*

Our experience is that this program will work for 80 to 90 percent of the people who follow it exactly. If you are one of the people for whom it does not work, read or reread the section on tough responders. You may need to do a more stringent elimination diet administered by a health professional (such programs usually involve hypoallergenic protein supplements and a pared-down diet such as lamb, rice, millet, and pears), or you could try some rare foods (see Appendix B). This entails eating foods you probably never normally eat.

- *What if I don't have an appetite?*

Eat more soups and stews. Try pureeing and heating all vegetables. It is often better to eat smaller portions throughout the day rather than the standard two or three large meals. Enzyme formulas such as Enzyme Harmony and Digestive Harmony will help pick up appetite for many people.

- *What if I fall off the program and my symptoms return?*

You may have a hunch as to what is causing your symptoms. Is it a sudden increase in stress or could it be a change in diet? I would suggest that you reread the relevant sections of this book and get back on the program.

- *What if the program doesn't work?*

You will have the satisfaction of knowing that you've given your best. This is why following the program exactly is so important. Unless you follow it exactly, you will never have a chance to see the program in action.

- *What if I'm cured during the preparation phase?*

Great. If you have no digestive problems while preparing to go on to the digestive clearing phase, you don't need to continue. Certainly many of the treatment principles (stress-reduction and exercise; reducing coffee, alcohol, and processed foods) help a significant number of people with digestive problems. I would suggest that you keep this up and eat with great variety.

- *What if I just can't complete the program?*

If you have noticed some benefits without finishing the program, please acknowledge yourself for trying and make a conscious note of the changes that seemed to help. If you have not yet tried Digestive Harmony, I urge you to try it. If you feel that you still have a long way to go, I suggest locating a holistic health professional who may be able to suggest vitamins or herbs that can help. For some people, it is much easier working with a practitioner. If you feel that you have received no benefit, you probably found yourself at a stressful period of your life, in which making changes was just not a possibility. If this is the case, I again urge you to visit a holistic health professional. If you are unable to make any diet changes at this time, at least maintain the stress-reduction and exercise part of the program.

- *What if I'm taking pharmaceutical drugs? Can I still do the program?*

If you have been taking the medication for several weeks, yes. If you have recently begun taking a medication, you should wait until you have been on it for several weeks. You should always discuss reducing or eliminating medication with your health professional.

- *My doctor says there's no science behind this. Who's right?*

Despite the best science in the world, many digestive problems are considered incurable. Medical science is particularly good at diagnosing conditions. It is not particularly good at creating health, which is the purpose of this book.

- *I followed the program as best as I could, but I saw little benefit. Why?*

Either you follow the program, or you don't. If you did the best you could, you need to redo weeks three and four of the program. Every day that you cheat means you are only fourteen days from completing the program.

Food Families

This section can be used especially during the reintroduction phase (weeks five and after). If you have allergies or intolerance to one of the mentioned foods, you may have reactions to foods in the same family. It also makes sense to investigate different preparation methods or varieties. For example, red apples/green apples, pesticide-free apples, or cooked apples, not raw, may make a big difference in your health.

*Foods with an asterisk can be considered for the rare foods diet.

PLANT CLASSIFICATION

APPLE
Apple Cider
Apple pectin
Juice
Pear
Quince

*Quince seed
  Vinegar

ARROWROOT
Arrowroot

ARUM
Dasheen
Malanga
Poi
*Taro
Yautia

BANANA
Banana
Plantain

BEECH
Beechnut
*Chestnut

BIRCH
Filbert
Hazelnut
Oil of birch

BORAGE
Borage
Comfrey

BRAZIL NUT
Brazil nut

BUCKWHEAT
Buckwheat
Rhubarb
Sorrel

CACTUS
Prickly pear
Tequila

CAPER
Capers

CASHEW
Cashew
Mango
Pistachio

CHINESE WATER
CHESTNUT
Chestnut, Chinese

CITRUS
Citron
Grapefruit
Kumquat
Lemon
Lime
Orange
Tangerine

COMPOSITE
Absinthe
Artichoke,
common
Celtuce
Chamomile
Chicory
Dandelion
Endive
Escarole
Goldenrod
Lettuce
Head
Leaf
*Jerusalem artichoke
Oyster plant
Ragweed and
pyrethrum, and
other related
inhalants
*Safflower
Sagebrush
Salsify

Sesame seed
Sunflower
Tarragon
Wormwood

EBONY
*Persimmon

FUNGI
Mushroom
Yeast

GINGER
Cardamom
Ginger
Turmeric

GINSENG
Ginseng

GOOSEBERRY
Currant
Gooseberry

GOOSEFOOT
Beet
Beet sugar
Chard
Lamb's quarters
Spinach
*Swiss chard
Thistle

GOURD
Cantaloupe
*Casaba

Christmas melon
Cucumber
Gherkin
Honeydew
Muskmelon
Persian melon
*Pumpkin
Squash
  Summer
  Winter
Romaine lettuce
Watermelon
Zucchini

GRAINS (CEREAL, GRASSES)
Bamboo shoots
Barley
Bran
Cane
Cane sugar
Cartose
"Cerelose"
Corn
Cornmeal
Corn oil
Cornstarch
Corn sugar
Corn syrup
Dextrose
"Dyno"
"Farina"
Flour
Glucose
Gluten
Graham

Grits
Hominy
Kafir
Malt
Maltose
Molasses
*Millet
Oats
Popcorn
Rice
Rum
Semolina flour
*Sorghum
  "Sweetose"
Triticale
Turbinado
Wheat
Whiskey/bourbon
Wheat germ
*Wild rice

GRAPE
Brandy (grape)
Champagne
Cream of tartar
Grape
Grape wine
Raisin
Vinegar

HEATH
Blueberry
Cranberry
Huckleberry
Wintergreen

HOLLY
Bearberry
*Maté (or yerba maté)
Pokeberry
Yaupon tea

HONEYSUCKLE
Elderberry

IRIS
Saffron

KELP
Algin

LAUREL
*Avocado
Bay leaf
Cinnamon
Sassafras

LEGUMES
Alfalfa
Black-eyed pea
Bush bean
Carob
Chick pea (garbanzo)
Green bean
Green pea
Jack bean
Kidney bean
Lentil
Licorice
Lima bean

Mung bean
Navy bean
Pea
Peanut
Peanut oil
Pinto bean
Senna
Soybean Flour
Soybean Lecithin
Soybean Oil
String bean
Tonka bean
Tragacanth gum

LILY
Aloe
Asparagus
Bermuda onion
Chive
Garlic
Leek
Onion
Sarsaparilla
Scallion
Yucca (cassava)

MACADAMIA
*Macadamia nut

MADDER
Coffee

MALLOW
Cotton seed
  Meal Oil
*Okra

MAPLE
Maple sugar
Maple syrup

MAY APPLE
May apple

MINT
Artichoke, Chinese
Basil
Horehound
Lavender
Marjoram
Mint
Oregano
Peppermint
Rosemary
Sage
Savory
Spearmint
Thyme

MISCELLANEOUS
Honey

MORNING GLORY FAMILY
Sweet potato

MULBERRY
Breadfruit
Fig
Hops
Mulberry

MUSTARD

(BRASSICA)
Broccoli
Brussels sprouts
Cabbage
Cauliflower
Celery cabbage
Collard
Colza shoot
Horseradish
Kale
Kohlrabi
Mustard
Radish
Rutabaga
Turnip
Watercress

MYRTLE
Allspice
Cloves
Guava
Paprika
Pimento

NIGHTSHADE
Belladonna
Eggplant
Ground cherry
Paprika (yellow)
Peppers
  Cayenne
  Chili
  Green
  Red
  Red sweet
Potato

Tobacco
Tomato

NUTMEG
Mace
Nutmeg

OAK
Chestnut

OLIVE
Black olive (ripe)
Green olive
Olive oil

ORCHID
Vanilla

PALM
Coconut
Date
Palm cabbage
Palm oil
Sago

PAPAL
Papain
*Papaya

**PARSLEY
(CARROT)**
Angelica
Anise
Caraway
Carrot
Celeriac

Celery
Celery seed
Chervil
Coriander
Cumin
Dill
Fennel
Lovage
Parsley
Parsnip
Water celery

PAWPAW
Pawpaw

PEPPER
Black pepper
White pepper

PINE
Juniper
Pine nut

PINEAPPLE
Pineapple

PLUM
Almond
Apricot
Cherry
  Sour
  Sweet
  Wild
Nectarine
Peach
Plum

Prune

POMEGRANATE
Pomegranate

POPPY
Poppy seed

PURSLANE
New Zealand
  spinach
Purslane

ROSE
Blackberry
Boysenberry
Dewberry
Loganberry
Raspberry
  Black
  Red
Strawberry
Youngberry

SAPODILLA
Chicle

SOAPBERRY
Litchi nut

SPURGE
*Tapioca

STERCULIA	TEA	Walnut
Cacao	Tea	Black
Caffeine		English
Chocolate	WALNUT	
Cocoa	Butternut	YAM
Cola	Hickory	Chinese potato
Karaya gum	Pecan	Yam
Kola bean		

ANIMAL CLASSIFICATION

AMPHIBIAN	Lobster	sugar)
*Frog	Prawn	*Lamb
	Shrimp	Lard
BIRD		Milk
Chicken	MAMMALS	*Moose
Chicken eggs	*Antelope	Mutton
Duck	Bacon	Pig (pork)
Duck eggs	Bear	*Rabbit (cottontail,
*Goose	Beaver	hare, jackrabbit)
Goose eggs	Beef (cattle)	*Reindeer
Grouse	Bison	Sheep
Guinea hen	Bovine	Squirrel
*Partridge	*Buffalo	Veal
Peacock	Butter	Whale
Pheasant	Caribou	
*Pigeon	Cheese	MOLLUSKS
Quail	Cow's milk	Abalone
*Squab	Deer	Cephalopods
Turkey	*Deer (venison)	Clam
Turkey eggs	Dolphin	Cockle
	*Elk	Gastropods
CRUSTACEANS	Gelatin (beef)	Mussel
Crab	*Goat	Octopus
Crayfish	Ham	Oyster
Decapods	Lactose (milk	Pelecypods

278

Quahog
Scallop
Snail
Squid

REPTILES
*Alligator
Rattlesnake
*Turtle

FISH (SALTWATER)
Albacore
Amberjack
American eel
*Anchovy
Barracuda
*Bluefish
Bonito
Butterfish
Cod (scrod)
*Codfish
Croaker
Cusk
Dab
Dolphin
Drum
Eel
*Flounder
*Grouper
Haddock
Hake
Halibut
*Herring
Jack
*Mackerel
Mahi mahi

Marlin
Menhaden
Mullet
Pilchard (sardine)
Plaice
Pollack
Pompano
Porgy
Red snapper
Rosefish
    (whitebait)
Sailfish
*Sea Bass
Sea herring
Sea trout
Scorpionfish
Shad
Silver perch
Skipjack
Sole
Spot
Swordfish
Tarpon
Tilefish
Tuna
Turbot
Weakfish (spotted
    sea trout)
Yellow jack

**FISH
(FRESHWATER)**
*Bass
Black bass species
Buffalofish
Bullhead

Carp
*Catfish species
Chub
Crappie
Croaker
Freshwater drum
Minnow
Muskellunge
Paddlefish
*Perch
Pickerel
Pike
Pike, northern
Salmon species
Sauger
Shad (roe)
Smelt
Sturgeon
Sturgeon (caviar)
Sucker
Sunfish species
Trout species
Walleyed pike
White perch
*Whitefish
Yellow perch

Appendix C

Common Acupuncture Points Used in the Treatment of Digestive Conditions

Manipulation of acupuncture points either through needling or acupressure can be very effective in treating digestive conditions. Practitioners may find the following guide helpful in selecting suitable points.

Symptom(s)	Points
Abdominal Bloating	S-25 *(Tianshu)*, S-36 *(Zusanli)*, Sp-6 *(Sanyinjiao)*, P-6 *(Neiguan)*, Co-6 *(Qihai)*, Ear-Liver Point
Appendicitis	M-LE-13 *(Lanweixue)*, S-25 *(Tianshu)*, S-36 *(Zusanli)*, S-37 *(Shangjuxu)*, LI-4 *(Hegu)*, LI-11 *(Quchi)*, Sp-8 *(Diji)*, Sp-9 *(Yinlingquan)*, Sp-10 *(Xuehai)*, Li-2 *(Xingjian)*, B-25 *(Dachangshu)*, B-54 *(Weizhong)*, TB-10 *(Tianjing)*, Ear-Shenmen, Ear-Sympathetic
Constipation	LI-4 *(Hegu)*, LI-11 *(Quchi)*, S-25 *(Tianshu)*, S-40 *(Fenglong)*, B-25 *(Dachangshu)*, Li-3 *(Taichong)*, TB-6 *(Zhigou)*, Ear-Large Intestine, Ear-Rectum; with weakness, add S-36 *(Zusanli)*, Sp-6 *(Sanyinjiao)*, Co-4 *(Guanyuan)*, Co-6 *(Qihai)*, B-20 *(Pishu)*, K-6 *(Zhaohai)*

Crohn's Disease and Colitis	S-21 *(Liangmen)*, S-25 *(Tianshu)*, S-29 *(Guilai)*, S-44 *(Neiting)*, Li-3 *(Taichong)*, H-7 *(Shenmen)*, LI-4 *(Hegu)*, P-6 *(Neiguan)*; with diarrhea, use LI-11 *(Quchi)*, S-44 *(Neiting)*, Sp-9 *(Yinlingquan)*; with weakness, add moxibustion at S-25 *(Tianshu)*, S-36 *(Zusanli)*, Co-6 *(Qihai)*, Co-12 *(Zhongwan)*; for accompanying symptoms such as diarrhea, constipation, stress, etc., see respective entries
Diarrhea	**Acute:** S-25 *(Tianshu)*, S-36 *(Zusanli)*, B-25 *(Dachangshu)*; with cold signs, add Co-6 *(Qihai)*, Co-12 *(Zhongwan)*, B-20 *(Pishu)*, B-23 *(Shenshu)*, Gv-4 *(Mingmen)*, Gv-20 *(Baihui)*, K-3 *(Taixi)*; for heat signs, use S-44 *(Neiting)*, Sp-9 *(Yinlingquan)*, LI-4 *(Hegu)*, salt moxibustion at navel **Chronic:** B-20 *(Pishu)*, Co-4 *(Guanyuan)*, Co-12 *(Zhongwan)*, Gv-20 *(Baihui)*, S-36 *(Zusanli)*, K-7 *(Fuliu)*, M-LE-1 *(Lineiting)*
Esophageal Reflux	P-6 *(Neiguan)*, S-36 *(Zusanli)*, Co-6 *(Qihai)*, Co-12 *(Zhongwan)*, Li-13 *(Zhangmen)*, B-17 *(Geshu)*, B-20 *(Pishu)*, B-21 *(Weishu)*, M-UE-16 *(Zhongkui)*; with cold signs, add Co-6 *(Qihai)*, B-20 *(Pishu)*
Food Poisoning	S-25 *(Tianshu)*, S-44 *(Neiting)*, Sp-6 *(Sanjiao)*, LI-4 *(Hegu)*, P-6 *(Neiguan)*, Co-6 *(Qihai)*, Co-12 *(Zhongwan)*
Heartburn	Co-12 *(Zhongwan)*, S-36 *(Zusanli)*, Ear-Heartburn
Hemorrhoids	B-30 *(Baihuanshu)*, B-35 *(Huiyang)*, B-54 *(Weizhong)*, B-56 *(Chengjin)*, B-57 *(Chengshan)*, G-20 *(Baihui)*, Ear-Rectum, Ear-*Shenmen*
Hepatitis	**Jaundice:** GB-34 *(Yanglingquan)*, Li-3 *(Taichong)*, Li-14 *(Qimen)*, B-18 *(Ganshu)*, B-19 *(Danshu)*, Gv-9 *(Zhiyang)*, Gv-14 *(Dazhui)*, TB-6 *(Zhigou)* **Chronic:** GB-34 *(Yanglingquan)*, Li-3 *(Taichong)*, B-18 *(Ganshu)*, B-19 *(Danshu)*, Sp-6 *(Sanyinjiao)*, Sp-9 *(Yinlingquan)*, S-36 *(Zusanli)*

Hiatal Hernia	Co-6 *(Qihai)*, Co-12 *(Zhongwan)*, Li-3 *(Taichong)*, S-25 *(Tianshu)*, S-36 *(Zusanli)*, S-41 *(Jiexi)*, P-6 *(Neiguan)*; with cold signs, add Co-12 *(Zhongwan)*, Co-6 *(Qihai)*
Hiccups	B-13 *(Feishu)*, B-14 *(Jueyinshu)*, B-17 *(Geshu)*, Co-17 *(Shanzhong)*, P-6 *(Neiguan)*, Co-6 *(Qihai)*, Co-22 *(Tiantu)*
Irritable Bowel Syndrome	LI-4 *(Hegu)*, LI-10 *(Shousanli)*, S-25 *(Tianshu)*, S-36 *(Zusanli)*, Sp-6 *(Sanyinjiao)*, Sp-9 *(Yinlingquan)*, Co-6 *(Qihai)*, Co-12 *(Zhongwan)*, B-23 *(Shenshu)*, Gv-20 *(Baihui)*; with cold signs, add Co-6 *(Qihai)*, Co-12 *(Zhongwan)*, S-25 *(Tianshu)*
Liver and Gallbladder Pain	M-LE-23 *(Dannangxue)*, GB-34 *(Yanglingquan)*, GB-40 *(Qiuxu)*, Li-3 *(Taichong)*, Li-14 *(Qimen)*, TB-6 *(Zhigou)*, P-6 *(Neiguan)*, B-18 *(Ganshu)*, B-19 *(Danshu)*, Ear-Shenmen, Ear-Liver
Lower Abdominal Pain	Sp-6 *(Sanyinjiao)*, S-25 *(Tianshu)*, S-29 *(Guilai)*, Co-4 *(Guanyuan)*, Co-6 *(Qihai)*, Co-17 *(Shanzhong)*, LI-4 *(Hegu)*, Li-3 *(Taichong)*; with cold signs, add Co-6 *(Qihai)*, Co-12 *(Zhongwan)*, S-36 *(Zusanli)*
Nausea	P-6 *(Neiguan)*, S-36 *(Zusanli)*, Ear-Nausea, Ear-Shenmen
Parasites	Co-6 *(Qihai)*, S-2 *(Sibai)*, S-21 *(Liangmen)*, S-36 *(Zusanli)*, Sp-6 *(Sanyinjiao)*, Sp-9 *(Yinlingquan)*, Sp-15 *(Daheng)*, GB-34 *(Yanglingquan)* **Cupping:** tender Back *Shu* points **Bloodlet:** M-UE-9 *(Sifeng)*, M-LE-34 *(Baichongwo)*
Stomach Pain	P-6 *(Neiguan)*, Sp-4 *(Gongsun)*, Sp-6 *(Sanyinjiao)*, Sp-9 *(Yinlingquan)*, S-24 *(Huaroumen)*, S-25 *(Tianshu)*, S-44 *(Neiting)*, Co-6 *(Tianshu)*, Co-10 *(Xiawan)*, Co-12 *(Zhongwan)*, Co-17 *(Shanzhong)*, TB-6 *(Zhigou)*, LI-4 *(Hegu)*, Li-3 *(Taichong)*, Li-14 *(Qimen)*, B-17 *(Geshu)*, Ear-Zero, Ear-*Shenmen*

Stress	K-3 *(Taixi)* -leave in for up to one hour, H-7 *(Shenmen)*, P-6 *(Neiguan)*, B-12 *(Fengmen)*, Co-14 *(Juque)*, S-36 *(Zusanli)*, M-HN-3 *(Yintang)*, N-HN-22 *(Anmian)*, Ear-*Shenmen*, Ear-Heart, Ear-Liver, Ear-Endocrine
Ulcer	Co-12 *(Zhongwan)*, S-21 *(Liangmen)*, S-36 *(Zusanli)*, B-17 *(Geshu)*, B-21 *(Weishu)*, P-6 *(Neiguan)*, LI-4 *(Hegu)*

Appendix D

Additional Formulas

Following are the formulas not elaborated on in Chapter Three, their applications, and ingredients.

Astra 18 Diet

Typical Applications: Weight loss; edema.

Chinese Therapeutic Actions: Clear dampness and phlegm, disperse Qi, tonify spleen Qi.

Ingredients: Astragalus (Huang Qi), Alisma (Zi Xie), Gardenia (Zhi Zi) Cyperus (Xiang Fu), Coix (Yi Yi Ren), Tang-keui (Dang Gui), White Peony (Bai Shao), White Atractylodes (Bai Zhu), Platycodon (Jie Geng), Sargassum (Hai Zao), Crategus (Shan Zha), Scute (Huang Qin), Laminaria (Kun Bu), Magnolia (Huo Po), Pinella (Ban Xia), citrus (Chen Pi).

Astra C

Typical Applications: Preventive for colds and flu.

Chinese Therapeutic Actions: Strengthen Wei Qi, relieve the surface.

Ingredients: Astragalus (Huang Qi), White Atractylodes (Bai Zhu), Siler (Fang Feng), Rose Hips, Acerola, Vitamin C (Ascorbic acid), Zinc Citrate.

Astra Essence

Typical Applications: General tonic; memory decrease, frequent urination

Chinese Therapeutic Actions: Tonify kidney essence, yin and yang.

Ingredients: Astragalus root and seed (Huang Qi and Sha Yuan Ji Zi), Ligustrum (Nu Zhen Zi),Hoshouwu (He Shou Wu), Lycium fruit (Gou Qi Zi), Rehmannia (Shu Di Huang), Eucommia (Du Zhong), Cuscuta (Tu Si Zi), Ginseng (Ren Shen), Tang kuei (Dang Gui),Cornus (Shan Zhu Yu).

Astra Isatis

Typical Applications: Protocols for: Chronic Fatigue Syndrome, HIV, Herpes.

Chinese Therapeutic Actions: Tonify Qi, yin and yang, clear phlegm and toxins.

Ingredients: Isatis extract (Da Qing Ye and Ban Lan Gen), Astragalus (Huang Qi), Bupleurum (Chai Hu), Laminaria (Kun Bu), Codonopsis (Dang Shen), Epimedium (Yin Yang Huo), Lycium fruit (Gou Qi Zi), Dioscorea (Shan Yao), Broussonetia (Chu Shi Zi), White Atractylodes (Bai Zhu), Licorice (Gan Cao).

Backbone

Typical Applications: Low back pain; bone repair; incontinence; impotence.

Chinese Therapeutic Actions: Tonify kidney, strengthen sinews and bones, remove blood stasis.

Ingredients: Eucommia (Du Zhong), Psoralea (Bu Gu Zhi), Woodwardia (Gou Ji), Cuscuta (Tu Si Zi), Cistanche (Rou Cong Rong), Rehmannia (Shu Di Huang), Tortoise shell from Chinemys Reevesii (Gui Ban), Cyathulae (Chuan Niu Xi), Acanthopanax (Wu Jia Pi), Tang-kuei tails (Dang Gui Wei), Dipsacus (Xu Duan), Carthamus (Hong Hua), Myrrh (Mo Yao), Cornus (Shan Zhu Yu).

Calm Spirit

Typical Applications: Stress, anger, anxiety, depression.

Chinese Therapeutic Actions: Nourish heart yin.

Ingredients: Taurine, Magnesium aspartate, Amylase, CereCalase, Protease, Catalase, alpha-Galactosidase, Lipase, Glucoamylase, Cellulase, Malt Diatase, Biota (Bai Zi Ren), White Peony (Bai Shao), Tang-kuei (Dang Gui), Fu Shen (Fu Shen), Polygala (Yuan Zhi), Zizyphus (Suan Zao Ren), Ophiopogon (Mai Men Dong), Codonopsis (Dang Shen), Amber (Hu Po).

Channel Flow

Typical Applications: Pain-relieving and relaxant; joint, muscle, abdominal and gynecological pain and cramping; headache, arthritis, and fibromyalgia.

Chinese Therapeutic Actions: Regulates Qi and blood, warms the channels.

Ingredients: Corydalis (Yan Hu Suo), Angelica (Bai Zhi), Peony (Bai Shao), Cinnamon twig (Gui Zhi), Tang-kuei (Dang Gui), Salvia (Dan Shen), Myrrh (Mo Yao), Frankincense (Ru Xiang), Licorice (Gan Cao).

Clear Heat

Typical Applications: Protocols for viral infections, hepatitis, HIV.

Chinese Therapeutic Actions: Clear internal heat and toxin.

Ingredients: Isatis Extract (Ban Lan Gen and Da Qing Ye), Oldenlandia (Bai Hua She She Cao), Lonicera (Jin Yin Hua), Prunella (Xia Ku Cao) Andrographis (Chuan Xin Lian), Laminaria (Kun Bu), Viola (Zi Hua Di Ding), Cordyceps (Dong Chong Xia Cao), Licorice (Gan Cao).

Clear Phlegm *(Wen Dan Tang)*

Therapeutic Applications: Phlegm disorders, expectorant, sedative, bronchitis, nausea, vomiting, dizziness.

Chinese Therapeutic Actions: Heat in gallbladder, phlegm in stomach, bitter taste in mouth, slight thirst

Ingredients: Pinellia (Ban Xia), Citrus Peel (Chen Pi), Poria (Fu Ling), Aurantium (Zhi Shi), Bamboo Shavings (Zhu Ru), Arisaema (Tian Nan Xing), Agastache (Huo Xiang), Acorus (Shi Chang Pu), Licorice (Gan Cao).

Clearing

Typical Applications: Chronic vaginal or urethral irritation; bladder infections.

Chinese Therapeutic Actions: Clear heat, tonify spleen, resolve dampness.

Ingredients: Lotus seed (Lian Zi), Ophiopogon (Mai Men Dong), Poria (Fu Ling),White ginseng (Bai Ren Shen), Plantago (Che Qian Zi), Scute (Huang Qin), Glehnia (Sha Shen), Smilax (Tu Fu Ling),Astragalus (Huang Qi), Lycium bark (Di Gu Pi), Moutan (Mu Dan Pi), Red Peony (Chi Shao), Licorice (Gan Cao).

Coptis Purge Fire

Typical Applications: UTI; herpes; intense local inflammation: eye, ear, throat; hives.

Chinese Therapeutic Actions: Purge fire and toxins, dry dampness.

Ingredients: Coptis (Huang Lian), Lophatherum (Dan Zhu Ye), Bupleurum (Chai Hu), Rehmannia (Sheng Di Huang), Tang Kuei (Dang Gui), White Peony (Bai Shao), Akebia (Mu Tong), Anemarrhena (Zhi Mu), Phellodendron (Huang Bai), Gentiana (Long Dan Cao), Alisma (Ze Xie), Plantago seed (Che Qian Zi), Scute (Huang Qin), Sophora (Ku Shen), Forsythia (Lian Qiao), Gardenia (Zhi Zi), Licorice (Gan Cao).

Drain Dampness

(Wu Ling San)

Typical Applications: Edema, difficulty in urination, sensation of heaviness.

Chinese Therapeutic Actions: Stagnation of water and dampness in the body, strengthen the spleen.

Ingredients: Alisma (Ze Xie), Poria (Fu Ling), Polyporus (Zhu Ling), Cinnamon twig (Gui Zhi), White Atractylodes (Bai Zhu).

Ease 2

Typical Applications: Neck, shoulder, muscle tension. GI disorders, loose stools.

Chinese Therapeutic Actions: Harmonize yang and Wei, move liver Qi.

Ingredients: Bupleurum (Chai Hu), Pueraria (Ge Gen), Pinellia (Ban Xia), Cinnamon (GuiZhi), White Peony (Bai Shao), Ginseng (Ren Shen), Scute (Huang Qin),Licorice (Gan Cao), Ginger (Gan Jiang).

Ease Plus

Typical Applications: Addiction withdrawal; anxiety; insomnia, constipation.

Chinese Therapeutic Actions: Sedate liver yang, calm Shen.

Ingredients: Calcium carbonate (Mu Li and Long Gu), Bupleurum (Chai Hu), Ginseng (Ren Shen), Ginger (Gan Jiang), Pinellia (Ban Xia), Scute (Huang Qin), Cinnamon (Gui Zhi), Rhubarb (Da Huang), Vladimiria souliei (Mu Xiang).

Enhance

Typical Applications: Protocols for HIV, CFS.

Chinese Therapeutic Actions: Tonify Qi, blood, and essence; clear heat and toxins.

Ingredients: Red Ganoderma (Ling Zhi), Isatis extract (Ban Lan Gen and Da Qing Ye), Spatholobus extract (Ji Xue Teng), Astragalus (Huang Qi), Tremella (Bai Mu Er), Andrographis (Chuan Xin Lian), Lonicera (Jin Yin Hua), Aquilaria (Chen Xiang), Epimedium (Yin Yang Huo), Oldenlandia (Bai Hua She She Cao), Cistanche (Rou Cong Rong), Lycium fruit (Gou Qi Zi), Laminaria (Kun Bu), Tang-kuei (Dang Gui), Hu-chang (Hu Chang), American Ginseng (Xi Yang Shen), Schizandra (Wu Wei Zi), Ligustrum (Nu Zhen Zi), White Atractylodes (Bai Zhu), Rehmannia (Shu Di Huang), Salvia (Dan Shen), Curcuma (Yu Jin), Viola (Zi Hua Di Ding), Citrus (Chen Pi), Peony (Bai Shao), Ho Show Wu (He Shou Wu), Eucommia (Du Zhong), Cardamon (Sha Ren), Licorice (Gan Cao).

GB-6

Typical Applications: Prevent gallbladder attacks, dissolve stones.

Chinese Therapeutic Actions: Clears stagnant Qi and damp heat from the liver and gallbladder.

Ingredients: Curcuma (Yu Jin), Corydalis (Yan Hu Suo), Taraxacum (Pu Gong Ying), Melia (Chuan Lian Zi), Ji Nei Jin (Ji Nei Jin), Salvia (Dan Shen).

Gentle Senna

Typical Applications: Constipation.

Chinese Therapeutic Actions: Clear excess heat, regulate the body's water content.

Ingredients: Microcos (Po Bu Ye), Lonicera (Jin Yin Hua), Senna (Fan Xie Ye), Prunus (Yu Li Ren), Pueraria flower (Ge Hua), Magnolia (Huo Po), Aurantium (Zhi Shi), Rhubarb (Da Huang).

Heavenly Water

Typical Applications: PMS, irregular menses, headache, emotional instability.

Chinese Therapeutic Actions: Relieve liver Qi and fire, tonify spleen Qi and heart blood.

Ingredients: Gotu Kola (Centella asiatica), Chaste Tree Berries (Viticus Agnus-castus), Passion flower (Passiflorae Incarnatae), Pseudostellaria (Tai Zi Shen), Scute (Huang Qin), Pinellia (Ban Xia), Poria (Fu Ling), White Peony (Bai Shao), Tang-kuei, (Dang Gui), Cyperus (Xiang Fu), Tricosanthes (Tian Hua Fen), Red Dates (Da Zao), Baked Licorice (Zhi Gan Cao), Citrus (Chen Pi), Blue Citrus (Qing Pi).

Marrow Plus

Typical Applications: Bone marrow suppression, anemia.

Chinese Therapeutic Actions: Vitalize and tonify blood.

Ingredients: Spatholobus (Ji Xue Teng), He-shou-wu (Ho Shou Wu), Salvia (Dan Shen), Codonopsis (Dang Shen), Astragalus (Huang Qi), Ligusticum (Chuan Xiong), Raw Rehmannia (Sheng Di Huang), Cooked Rehmannia (Shu Di Huang), Lycium (Gou Qi Zi), Tang-kuei (Dang Gui), Lotus Seed (Lian Zi), Citrus (Chen Pi), Red Date Extract (Da Zao), Oryza (Gu Ya), Gelatinum (E Jiao).

Mobility 2

Typical Applications: Arthritis, gout, sciatica, lumbago.

Chinese Therapeutic Actions: Dispel damp cold, warm and vitalize blood.

Ingredients: Red Peony (Chi Shao), Tang-kuei (Dang Gui), Ligusticum (Chuan Xiong), Rehmannia (Shu Di Huang), Persica (Tao Ren), White Atractylodes (Bai Zhu), Poria (Fu Ling), Citrus (Chin Pi), Siler (Fang Feng), Vitex (Man Jing Zi), Gentiana (Long Dan Cao), Achyranthes (Niu Xi), Chiang-huo (Qiang Huo), Clematis (Wei Ling Xian), Ginger (Gan Jiang), Angelica (Bai Zhi), Licorice (Gan Cao).

Mobility 3

Typical Applications: Arthritis, headache, malaise due to exposure to wind, cold, dampness, arthritis.

Chinese Therapeutic Actions: Tonify and Invigorate blood, dispel: cold, wind, dampness.

Ingredients: Kirin Ginseng (Ji Ling Shen),Cinnamon Twig (Gui Zhi), Rehmannia (Shu Di Huang), Ho-shou-wu (He Shou Wu), Loranthus (Sang Ji Sheng), Tang-kuei (Dang Gui), Cistanche (Rou Cong Rong), Ardisia Gigantifolia (Zou Ma Tai), Chiang-huo (Qiang Huo), Angelica (Du Huo), Tienchi (San Qi), Spatholobus (Ji Xue Teng), Tinospora (Shen Jin Teng), Chaenomelis (Mu Gua), Achyranthes (Niu Xi), Ginger (Gan Jiang).

Nine Flavor Tea

Typical Applications: Diabetes, sore throat, tidal fever, wasting/thirsting syndrome.

Chinese Therapeutic Actions: Tonify kidney and liver yin, clear stomach heat.

Ingredients: Rehmannia (Sheng Di Huang), Dioscorea (Shan Yao), Poria (Fu Ling), Cornus (Shan Zhu Yu), Moutan (Mu Dan Pi), Alisma (Zi Xie), Scrophularia (Xuan Shen), Glehnia (Sha Shen), Ophiopogon (Mai Men Dong).

PB 8

Typical Applications: Restore healthy bacteria.

Ingredients: L acidophilus, L plantarum, L bulgaricus, L casei, S thermophilus, B bifidum, S faecicim, B infantis.

Power Mushrooms

Typical Applications: Immune enhancement, boost energy.

Chinese Therapeutic Actions: Tonify Qi.

Ingredients: Red Ganoderma (Rei Shi; Ling Zhi), Tremella (Bai Mu Er), Poria (Fu Ling), Polyporus (Zhu Ling).

Quercenol

Typical Applications: Antioxidant.

Ingredients (2 tablets): Quercetin (400 mg), Silybum marianum (250 mg), Proanthocyanidins (125 mg), Green tea polyphenols (150 mg), Mixed carotenoids (30 mg), Vitamin E (300 IU), Vitamin C (500 mg), Zinc (10 mg), Selenium (100 mcg).

Regeneration

Typical Applications: Enhances the immune system, used as an adjunct to surgery, chemotherapy, radiation therapy.

Chinese Therapeutic Actions: Strengthens the body, clears toxins, stops pain

Ingredients: Kirin Ginseng (Jilin Shen), Tang-kuei (Dang Gui), Akebia fruit (Ba Yue Zha), Soarganium (San Leng), Zedoaria (E Zhu), Tienchi (San Qi), Gentiana (Long Dan Cao), Scute (Huang Qin), Qin Jiao, Persica (Tao Ren), Moutan (Mu Dan Pi), White Peony (Bai Shao).

Resinall E Tabs

Typical Applications: Treats pain and swelling due to traumatic injuries—sprains, strains, contusions, fractures, broken bones, torn sinews, bleeding, bruising, lacerations.

Chinese Therapeutic Actions: Promotes tissue regeneration, activates blood, stops bleeding.

Ingredients: *Enzymes:* Bromelain 100 mg, Rutin 100 mg, Papain 50 mg, Trypsin 50 mg, Chymotrypsin 100 mcg, Dragon's Blood (Xue Jie), Tienchi (San Qi), Catechu (Er Cha), Corydalis (Yan Hu Suo), Carthamus (Hong Hua), Myrrh (MoYao), Frankincense (Ru Xiang), Borneol (Bing Pian).

Resinall K

Typical Applications: Pain/swelling of traumatic injury, chronic fixed pain.

Chinese Therapeutic Actions: Relieve blood stagnation.

Ingredients: Dragon's blood (Xue Jie), Tienchi (San Qi), Catechu (Er Cha), Corydalis (Yan Hu Suo), Carthamus (Hong Hua), Myrrh (Mo Yao), Frankincense (Ru Xiang), Borneol (Bing Pian), Alcohol, Glycerin.

Sea-Q

Typical Applications: General tonic, anti-arthritic, anti-inflammatory, used for impotence.

Chinese Therapeutic Actions: Tonifies the liver/kidney, nourishes the blood, relieves swelling.

Ingredients: Sea Cucumber (Microchele nobilis, Hai Shen), Sargassum (Hai Zhao).

Shen-Gem

Typical Applications: Insomnia, nervousness, palpitations.

Chinese Therapeutic Actions: Tonify spleen Qi and heart blood.

Ingredients: Ginseng (Ren Shen), Poria (Fu Ling), White Atractylodes (Bai Zhu), Zizyphus (Suan Zao Ren), Astragalus (Huang Qi), Tang-kuei (Dang Gui), Salvia (Dan Shen), Amber (Hu Po), Polygala (Yuan Zhi), Longan (Long Yan Rou), Vladimiria Souliei (Mu Xiang), Ginger (Gan Jiang), Licorice (Gan Cao), Cardamon (Sha Ren).

Shu Gan

Typical Applications: Gynecology, food allergies, nausea, burping, vomiting and regurgitation associated with hyperacidity, anorexia, bulimia.

Chinese Therapeutic Actions: Liver Qi stagnation, aids digestion, relieves pain in the middle burner.

Ingredients: Curcuma tuber (Yu Jin), Aquilaria wood (Chen Xiang), Corydalis root (Yan Hu Suo), Vladimiria Souliei (Mu Xiang), Nutmeg seed (Rou Dou Kou), White Peony root (Bai Shao), Citrus fruit (Zhi Ke), Citrus peel (Chen Pi), Cardamon fruit (Sha Ren), Magnolia bark (Hou Po), Cypress rhizome (Xiang Fu), Licorice root (Gan Cao), Moutan root (Mu Dan Pi), Immature Citrus Peel (Qing Pi), Sandalwood (Tan Xiang).

Tremella and American Ginseng

Typical Applications: Chronic viral syndromes.

Chinese Therapeutic Actions: Tonifies yin, Qi, blood, essence; strengthens marrow, Wei Qi, spleen/stomach, lungs, kidney; clears heat and toxin.

Ingredients: Tremella (Bai Mu Er), American Ginseng (Xi Yang Shen), Astragalus (Huang Qi), Schizandra (Wu Wei Zi), Raw Rehmannia (Sheng Di Huang), Lycium cortex (Gou Qi Zi), Lycium bark (Di Gu Pi), Isatis extract (Ban Lan Gen/Da Qing Ye), Ophiopogon (Mai Men Dong), Lonicera (Jin Yin Hua), Viola (Zi Hua Di Ding), Red Ganoderma (Ling Zhi), Cuscuta (Tu Si Zi), Ephemerantha (You Gua Shi Hua), Spatholobus (Ji Xue Teng), Ligustrum (Nu Zhen Zi), Glehnia (Sha Shan), Tang-keui (Dang Gui), Tortoise shell from Chinemys reevesii (Gui Ban), Epimedium (Yin Yang Huo), Citrus (Chen Pi), Curcuma (Yu Jin), Licorice (Gan Cao), Cardamon (Sha Ren).

Vagistatin

Typical Applications: Cervical dysplasia, HPV, Candidiasis.

Chinese Therapeutic Actions: Dispel toxic heat, damp heat.

Ingredients: Isatis extract (Ban Lan Gen and Da QingYe), Phellodendron (Huang Bai), Salvia (Dan Shen), Artemesia (Qing Hao), Houttuynia (Yu Xing Cao), Cnidium fruit (She Chuang Zi), Agrimony (Xian He Cao).

Woman's Balance

Typical Applications: PMS, bloating, breast swelling, menstrual irregularity.

Chinese Therapeutic Actions: Move liver Qi, harmonize liver and spleen.

Ingredients: Bupleurum (Chai Hu), Tang-kuei (Dang Gui), White Peony (Bai Shao), Salvia (Dan Shen), Poria (Fu Ling), White Atractylodes (Bai Zhu), Cyperus (Xiang Fu), Citrus (Chen Pi), Moutan (Mu Dan Pi), Gardenia (Zhi Zi), Ginger (Gan Jiang), Licorice (Gan Cao).

Appendix E

Resource Guide

The following are organizations or agencies that offer information and support to persons with digestive conditions.

For further information, a list of practitioners in your area who recommend herbs, and/or information about seminars or our upcoming newsletter, write to the author:

Andrew Gaeddert

c/o Get Well Clinic
8001A Capwell Drive
Oakland, CA 94621
Telephone: 510-635-9778
Fax: 510-639-9140
E-mail: info@getwellfoundation.org

American Celiac Society

Dietary Support Coalition
58 Musano Court
West Orange, NJ 07052
Telephone: 973-325-8837

American Liver Foundation

1425 Pompton Avenue
Cedar Grove, NJ 07009
Telephone: 800-223-0179

Center for Ulcer Research and Education Foundation

P.O. Box 84513
Los Angeles, CA 90073
Telephone: 213-825-5091

Crohn's and Colitis Foundation of America

444 Park Avenue South
New York, NY 10016
Telephone: 212-685-3440; 800-343-3637

Gluten Intolerance Group of America

P.O. Box 23053
Seattle, WA 98102
Telephone: 206-325-6980; 518-489-0972

Intestinal Disease Foundation, Inc.

1323 Forbes Avenue, Suite 200
Pittsburgh, PA 15219
Telephone: 412-261-5888

National Cancer Institute

Cancer Information Service
Telephone: 800-4-CANCER
http://rex.nci.nih.gov

National Digestive Disease Information Clearinghouse

P.O. Box NDDIC
9000 Rockville Pike
Bethesda, MD 20892
Telephone: 301-654-3810

Oley Foundation for Home Parenteral and Enteral Nutrition

214 Hun Memorial
Albany Medical Center
Albany, NY 12208
Telephone: 800-776-OLEY

United Ostomy Association

36 Executive Park, Suite 120
Irvine, CA 92714
Telephone: 714-660-8624; 800-826-0826

References

Balch, James, and Phyllis Balch. *Prescription for Nutritional Healing.* Garden City Park, NY: Avery Publishing Group, 1993.

Brostoff, Jonathan, and Linda Gamlin. *The Complete Guide to Food Allergy and Intolerance.* New York, NY: Crown, 1989.

Castleman, Michael. *The Healing Herbs.* New York, NY: Bantam, 1995.

Chaitow, Leon, and Natasha Trenev. *Probiotics.* London: Thorsons, 1990.

Crook, William G. *The Yeast Connection and the Woman.* Jackson, TN: Professional Books, 1995.

Fisher, Jeffrey A. *The Plague Makers.* New York, NY: Simon and Schuster, 1994.

Fung, Fung, and John Fung. *Sixty Years in Search of Cures.* Dublin, CA: Get Well Foundation, 1994.

Gaeddert, Andrew. *Chinese Herbs in the Western Clinic.* Dublin, CA: Get Well Foundation, 1994.

Gottschall, Elaine. *Food and the Gut Reaction.* Kirkton, Ontario: The Kirkton Press, 1986.

Graedon, Joe, and Teresa Graedon. *Dead Drug Interactions: The People's Pharmacy Guide.* New York, NY: St. Martin's Press, 1995.

Greenwood, Jan K. *The IBD Nutrition Book.* New York, NY: John Wiley and Sons, 1992.

Guillory, Gerrard. *IBS: A Doctor's Plan for Chronic Digestive Troubles: The Definitive Guide to Prevention and Relief.* Point Roberts, WA: Hartley and Marks, 1991.

Hoffman, David. *The New Holistic Herbal.* Rockport, MA: Element Books, 1983.

Hoffman, Ronald. *7 Weeks to a Settled Stomach.* New York, NY: Pocket Books, 1990.

Janowitz, Henry D. *Indigestion: Living Better with Upper Intestinal Problems, From Heartburn to Ulcers and Gallstones.* New York, NY: Oxford University Press, 1992.

———. *Your Gut Feeling: A Complete Guide to Living Better with Intestinal Problems.* New York, NY: Oxford University Pres, 1987.

Kaminski, Patricia, and Richard Katz. *Flower Essence Repertory.* Nevada City, CA: Flower Essence Society, 1994.

Levy, Stuart B. *The Antibiotic Paradox.* New York, NY: Plenum, 1992.

Margolis, Simeon, and the Editors of *The Johns Hopkins Medical Letter: Health After 50. Johns Hopkins Symptoms and Remedies.* New York, NY: Rebus, 1995.

Murray, Michael, and Joseph Pizzorno. *Encyclopedia of Natural Medicine.* Revised 2nd ed. Rocklin, CA: Prima, 1996.

National Foundation for Ileitis and Colitis. *The Crohn's Disease and Ulcerative Colitis Fact Book.* New York, NY: Macmillan, 1983.

Nicol, Rosemary. *Irritable Bowel Syndrome: A Natural Approach.* Berkeley, CA: Ulysses Press, 1995.

Scala, James. *Eating Right for a Bad Gut.* New York, NY: Plume Books, 1992.

Schuster, Marvin M., and Jacqueline Wehmueller. *Keeping Control*. Baltimore, MD: The Johns Hopkins University Press, 1994.

Shannon, Margaret T., Carolyn L. Stang, and Billie Ann Wilson. *Nurses Drug Guide, 1998*. Stamford, CT: Appleton and Lange, 1998.

Shimberg, Elaine Fantle. *Relief from IBS*. New York, NY: Ballantine Books, 1991.

Thompson, W. Grant. *Gut Reactions*. New York, NY: Plenum, 1989.

——. *The Angry Gut*. New York, NY: Plenum, 1993.

Trickett, Shirley. *Irritable Bowel Syndrome and Diverticulosis*. London: Thorsons, 1990.

Valnet, Jean. *The Practice of Aromatherapy*. New York, NY: Destiny Books, 1980.

Weiss, Rudolf Fritz. *Herbal Medicine*. Beaconsfield, England: Beaconsfield Publishers, 1988.

Xu, Xiangcai. *The English-Chinese Encyclopedia of Practical Traditional Chinese Medicine*. Beijing: Higher Education Press, 1989.

Yang, Shou-Zhong, and Li Jian-Yong. *Li Dong-Yuan's Treatise of the Spleen and Stomach*. Boulder, CO: Blue Poppy Press, 1993.

Index

Books Available
from Get Well Foundation

Healing Immune Disorders

by Andrew Gaeddert ISBN 1-55643-604-1 $18.95

Healing Immune Disorders contains the latest scientific research on herbs and supplements and protocols for all major immune and autoimmune conditions. Whether you are a patient or a professional, you will be able to benefit from the advice in this book.

Digestive Health Now

by Andrew Gaeddert ISBN 1-55643-426-6 $12.95

Digestive Health NOW explains a four-week program that can be completed in your home using a meal plan, recipes, and stress relieving techniques. Included are real-life stories of people who have been able to reduce or eliminate medication, and achieve an understanding of what causes symptoms and how to prevent them.

Healing Skin Disorders

by Andrew Gaeddert ISBN 1-55643-452-9 $15.95

Filled with self-help strategies, treatment protocols, and case studies for all major skin disorders, this book is designed for the professional as well as the layperson. Dietary advice, acupuncture points, herbs, and nutritional supplements make this the most complete book of its kind.

Healing Digestive Disorders

by Andrew Gaeddert   ISBN 1-55643-743-4 $18.95

This revised third edition by herbalist Andrew Gaeddert lists self-help strategies, treatment protocols, and case studies for all major digestive disorders. Designed for the professional as well as the layperson, *Healing Digestive Disorders* also contains the story of how the author conquered Crohn's disease, a recommended meal plan, workbook section, and acupuncture points.

Chinese Herbs in the Western Clinic

by Andrew Gaeddert   ISBN 0-96382-850-9 $15.95

Chinese Herbs in the Western Clinic recommends formulas by a variety of manufacturers that have been successfully used with thousands of American patients suffering from immune, digestive, gynecological, respiratory disorders, and other commonly seen complaints such as allergies, anxiety, arthritis, back pain, headaches, injury, insomnia and stress. Disorders are alphabetized by Western conditions and indexed by traditional Chinese medical terminology for easy reference while patients are in the office. This book is designed for practitioners.

Sixty Years in Search of Cures

by Dr. Fung Fung and John Fung   ISBN 0-96382-851-7 $15.95

Sixty years in Search of Cures is the autobiography of one of the world's most experienced herbalists, Dr. Fung Fung, who routinely saw 100 to 150 patients per day working in a hospital clinic. This master practitioner with experience in Canton, Hong Kong, Vietnam, and San Francisco, reveals important dietary and lifestyle habits for the general public and herbal prescriptions for the professional herbalist.

Send check or money order payable to Get Well. Include $2.00 per book shipping and handling. California residents add CA sales tax of 8.75% per book. Please be sure to write your name and address clearly, and to specify the titles and quantities of each book you want. Allow 4 weeks for delivery.

For trade, bookstore, and wholesale inquiries, contact North Atlantic Books, P.O. Box 12327, Berkeley, CA 94712.

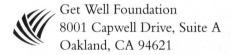 Get Well Foundation
8001 Capwell Drive, Suite A
Oakland, CA 94621

About the Author

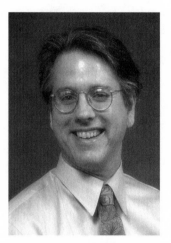

Andrew Gaeddert suffered from Crohn's disease and IBS. His search for therapies to treat his own symptoms led to the discovery of techniques that have made it possible for him to help thousands of other people. Mr. Gaeddert has studied nutrition, herbology, and Chinese medicine with masters of herbal medicine from the United States and China. He has been on the protocol team of several scientific studies sponsored by the NIH Office of Alternative Medicine and the University of California. He has lectured at Columbia University, University of San Francisco, Canadian College of Oriental medicine, and other colleges across the United States. His students have included medical doctors, acupuncturists, herbalists, and other professionals. Mr. Gaeddert is also the author of *Chinese Herbs in the Western Clinic, Healing Skin Disorders,* and *Healing Immune Disorders.* He is the president of Health Concerns in Oakland, California, whose purpose is to help millions of Americans suffering from chronic, stress-related, and immune-compromised conditions.